BRUTE FORCE
BEGINNER'S STRENGTH SYSTEM

KEN GACK 'THE RIPPER'

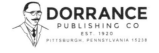

DORRANCE
PUBLISHING CO
EST. 1920
PITTSBURGH, PENNSYLVANIA 15238

Dorrance Publishing Co
585 Alpha Drive
Pittsburgh, PA 15238
Visit our website at *www.dorrancebookstore.com*

ISBN: 978-1-6470-2519-9
eISBN: 978-1-6470-2693-6

CONTENTS

FOREWORD AND ACKNOWLEDGMENTS

Powerlifting has been my passion my entire adult life. It has given me physical strength, but also built self-confidence and given me a personal strength that has grown to permeate every facet of my life. It has taken me, literally, around the world and introduced me to a new family in the powerlifting community.

I would like to thank my friends and family for supporting this project. My wife has been incredibly patient, supporting my lifelong and passionate relationship with the powerlifting lifestyle that has culminated in the creation of this book. Without your support during the hours away for training every week and more hours with my nose in the screen and fingers on the keyboard, this project would never have happened. Thank you to the close friends who have kept me sane and focused. I must also thank my sister for kicking my ass into actually sitting down with pen and paper to write this book.

Sitting down with a keyboard. Who writes by hand anymore? Savages!

I would like to thank all the lifters I have coached over the years. Your patience with my experiments has been an integral ingredient in developing this book and training system. A special thanks to those of you who have been with me since the very beginning, and still eagerly attack my new experiments.

Also, I'd like to thank the lifting clubs I've been a part of. The Ramstein Powerlifting Club and coach Gene Bell, who gave me my powerlifting start; my current club, Team Phoinix, coach Kevin Stewart, anti-coach Mike/Todd, and all the team members who have helped me hone my skills and kept me from dying.

When I began lifting several lifetimes ago, there were very few good sources of lifting information for the average gym rat - my introduction to the weight room at Lackland Air Force Base preceded the Internet and Instagram. I watched, I tried, and I learned. Occasionally I picked up a bodybuilding mag and devoured the one or two gratuitous strength articles they'd tossed in.

After several years of trial and error and error and error, I had the fortune to be adopted onto Gene Bell's (one of powerlifting's all-time greats) powerlifting teams. Gene introduced me to powerlifting and ignited my passion for the platform. He introduced me to periodized training concepts and taught me the critical importance of mastering lifting technique. In one squat session, for example, he tweaked my squat technique and added 50lbs to my max.

Today the landscape is the polar opposite. The internet and social media are chock full of lifting information and there are myriads of tools and techniques at your fingertips. Your challenge today is weeding through the chaff for those precious nuggets of good information. You are tasked with sorting the good information for what is most applicable to you and your lifting situation and goals.

Even with this abundance of data, there is a relatively small amount of new and original content. Much of what you find out there in the Internet wild is built on and expands an existing base. We find new ways to use and repackage it. That is a good thing.

Brute Force Beginner's Strength System, referred to as 'the System' throughout this book, builds on a foundation set in a couple important strength and powerlifting approaches:

- Periodization
- Reactive Training System's (RTS) autoregulation approaches and emerging strategies concepts

How these approaches have been woven into the System is described in chapter 2, the Training Approach. Having spent over thirty years building and expanding my lifting toolbox, there are many other influences on my approach, but these are the ones that have had the greatest impact. My hope is that you can use the System to build your toolbox as well.

LIABILITY STATEMENT

It is important to understand that any type of physical activity inherently involves some risk. Before embarking on any new physical training regimen, it is important to make sure you can perform the activities properly and safely. Please consult your physician before starting this, or any new training program. Consult them also if your physical condition or preparedness changes at any point during the execution of the program.

The intent of this program is to develop incredible physical strength while minimizing the risk of injury. However, any time you get under the bar there is a risk that bad things happen. You, the reader, accept the risk and the liability for any injuries experienced while following this program. You also reap the monumental rewards that come with accepting that risk (incredible physical strength).

Now that the necessary words are out of the way, let's get under the bar!

Chapter 1

BACKGROUND AND CONCEPT

"Life's Too Short to be Small"
Or weak.

Who did I write this for?

I developed the System primarily for relatively new, novice lifters. If you have less than two years under the bar, you likely have significant potential for 'new lifter gains'. Your strength can progress relatively quickly. It is vitally important during this this phase to create good training habits, build solid technique and develop the broad foundation in strength you will continue to build on throughout your lifting career (which hopefully spans many decades).

Note: If you are a novice lifter, I encourage you to review technique for lifts you perform in the System. I have a set of technique primers for the most important lifts in my Book of Techniques at https://bruteforcestrength/bfs-book-of-techniques/ . I encourage intermediate and experienced lifters alike to review lift techniques from time to time to find ways to fine tune your technique.

Although created for novice lifters, the System can be effectively leveraged by intermediate to experienced lifters whose current goal is to rebuild or expand their strength foundation. It also includes tips and tools that lifters of all experience levels may find useful.

What is the System based on?

Before getting into any programming details, there are some fundamental training concepts that you should understand. These concepts affect training regardless what your end goal is, be it strength and power, hypertrophy, endurance, or fitness and body composition.

- *Law of Individual Differences*: Every person is different. There are an unlimited number of differences that may affect an individual's training – body dimensions, muscle fiber composition, muscle attachment points, training history, training goals, even an individual's personality. Because we are all unique individuals, there is no one size fits all with respect to training. Some important variables I try to address with this program include:
  - Body mechanics: Everyone is built differently – height, weight, build, arm and leg length, the list can go on. These differences affect your training. They can impact how you set up for a lift, exercise selection, they may even dictate where your weak points lie.
  - Strengths and Weaknesses: Training history, past injuries, body mechanics and many other factors dictate where your strengths and weaknesses lie. Understanding this and planning to mitigate your weaknesses while emphasizing your strengths is necessary to maximize your performance.
  - Responses to different stimulus: People respond to training differently. Some people excel with very high volume, some people get bored quickly without training variety. Failing to take this into account will limit a program's success.

  A good program is tailored not only to a lifter's strengths, weaknesses, and mechanics, but also to their preferences. This concept is a primary reason I have never been a fan of pre-built workouts promoted by fitness 'experts' or inflexible training templates.

- *Volume and intensity*: Volume refers to the number of sets and reps in a program, intensity refers to the weights used relative to your strength level. There are training ranges that favor hypertrophy versus strength or power versus other training goals.

  Much of the training in the System hovers in the strength training range. The final training block starts to dip into the power training range, and accessory work dips into the hypertrophy range. The purpose of this mix is to build a broad, well-balanced muscular and strength foundation.

- *Autoregulation*: Autoregulation is a fundamental training principle I have borrowed from Reactive Training Systems. It is the process of increasing the intensity on your strong days and reducing the intensity on your off days. We all know that some days you go to the gym ready to conquer the world, and other days you are dragging. Basing your training on eighty percent of last July's 1RM is just not as effective as basing it on how effectively you're lifting *today*.

  On the strong days, autoregulation relaxes the reigns, lets you push harder. Autoregulation takes advantage of that heightened energy. On off days it allows you to pull back a bit, get what you can, and finish your training plan without killing yourself to hit an arbitrary number.

  Note: autoregulation is *not* a license to max out in every training session.

- *Progressive Overload*: This concept is quite simple, to get stronger, you must lift more weight.

  With the System, the autoregulation mechanism allows you to adjust for your strength level on any given day (if you feel stronger you lift heavier, if you're tired and beat up, you lift lighter). Over the course of the program, however, the periodization component facilitates handling progressively heavier loads.

- *The body's adaptation to stimuli*: Over time, the body begins to adapt to the stimuli presented. This is how you get stronger. If a set of squats nearly kills you, your body adapts and grows stronger (adding muscle mass, improving CNS efficiency, strengthening tendons, etc.) so that the next time you can more readily handle it. These adaptations are what make progressive overload effective and necessary. As your body gets stronger, you need to challenge it harder.

  That said, simple progressive overload only works to an extent. At some point, the body's adaptation slows in response to simple changes in intensity. To continue to grow stronger, other components of your training must change as well. Within the System, the overall training stimulus is modified from block to block, as described in chapter 2, to keep the body adapting and getting stronger.

- *Technical mastery*: Lifting heavy weights is a skill. To be good at it, you need to practice. Although the training changes as you progress through the System, continuously stimulating body adaptations, key lifting patterns remain constant throughout the program. You will stick with your primary lifts throughout the program to build your technical mastery of those lifts.

Why did I write this book?
Don't get me wrong, there are many good training programs out there. For beginners who are interested in building incredible strength, my preference has leaned toward those based on a 5x5 structure. 5x5 is a good meat and potatoes strength building approach. It balances volume and intensity for strength gains. With the System, I am trying to harness the strength of the 5x approaches, and enhance it with training techniques I've found quite effective:

- Periodization
- Autoregulation
- Reactive Training Systems' Emerging Strategies

Some key goals that I emphasize in my coaching and throughout this book are:

- Heavy use of major compound lifts in the four lifting domains: Lower Body Push (squats), Upper Body Push (bench press and overhead press), Lower Body Pull (deadlifts), Upper Body Pull (rows and pull-ups).
- Creating a balanced program that doesn't neglect any major muscular systems. This means including accessory work to bring up secondary and stabilizer muscle groups that may be lacking.
- Basing your training intensity on your strength levels *today*, not where you were three years ago when you hit your all time max or some arbitrary future goal.

- Emphasis on technical mastery. All lifts are to be performed with technical competence before moving on. If you train with me in person, you may hear this a lot: "that rep didn't count, do it again"

What you should take away from the System:

- *Get Stronger*: The fundamental purpose of the System, after all, is to get stronger. Keep in mind that there are more aspects to strength than the number on the bar. Does the bar move faster at the same weight? Has your technique improved at all weights? Are you completing the lifts without cheating (hitting depth on squats, controlling the bar without bouncing off your chest in the bench press)?
- *Technical Mastery*: Mastery may be a misnomer. After lifting for thirty years, I still try to find ways to improve the technique on my lifts. But as you build your strength foundation, you should master the lifts to the degree that you can lift near max weights without significant technique flaws.
- *Build a Broad Physical Foundation*: The Egyptian pyramids were built 4,500 years ago and still stand proudly. Build your strength foundation in the same way, developing strength that will last a lifetime. Train all your muscle systems in balance. Build tendon strength and bone density to support max effort loads over time. Don't rush the weights before your muscular and skeletal systems have been built to handle it – stacking blocks precariously on top of each other. Stack them instead of upon a solid, broad foundation.
- *Strengthen Weaknesses and Rehab Injuries*: As you assess your strength in the various lifts, also work to identify where your weaknesses lie. Audit current and historic injuries and take them into account as you plan future training. Failure to address them as you build strength can increase your chance of further injury and setbacks. Addressing them properly can build a more powerful, stable strength foundation, taking your lifts to new levels.

How to use this book:
Some of you are not going to read this book cover to cover (you know who you are). I have laid it out so for those of you who are ready, you can jump in

and start lifting. The appendices are structured to be a reference to the System. Use them to understand the System's structure, and how to use the tools and templates that I've included to make your training highly effective.

For those who do read cover to cover, I hope you find it informative and entertaining!

Chapter 2

TRAINING APPROACH

"Hope is not a strategy"

How do I apply these basic concepts?
In chapter 1, I discussed some fundamental strength building concepts upon which the System is based. In this chapter I'll review how I apply them in a cohesive, balanced manner. Here is a quick overview:

- Weakness assessment: You begin your training with an assessment. Although the primary goal is to define your training's starting point, you'll also use this assessment to identify weak points. Some things to consider when assessing your weaknesses:
  - What are the weak points in your range of motion?
  - At what point in the lift does form break down?
  - What are your technique issues?
  - Do you have any past or current injuries that affect your lifts?

  Using this knowledge, tailor your program to strengthen areas of weakness. Focusing on weaknesses and technique issues will have a major impact on not only your strength levels, but also your resistance to injury. To help you with this, in Appendix D I have included a robust set of recommendations for strengthening weaknesses and correcting technique flaws.

- Periodization theories: Periodization theories were introduced by the Russians in the 60s. Variations of this approach has successfully trained generations of strength athletes. At its most basic level, the concept of periodization is that as you progress through the program you increase the weight and decrease the volume. For example, it might look something like:

  Block 1: 5x5 @ 70%
  Block 2: 5x4 @ 75%
  Block 3: 5x3 @ 80%

This approach helps address the body's adaptation to stimuli by changing the volume and intensity at regular intervals. It also facilitates progressive overload by increasing the intensity with each block.

In the System, I modify the rigid structure most periodization schemes use and allow you to adapt to your current and emerging capabilities (leveraging RTS' Emerging Strategies theories). You will base each training block on your current estimated strength levels, not your 1RM from some past training cycle, nor some arbitrary training goal. It also allows for adjustment based on your daily capabilities as discussed below under auto-regulation. By relaxing the rigid periodization structure, this flexibility enhances the strengths of the periodization approach and helps you maximize your potential in each training session.

- Auto-regulation: On any given day your strength level, training motivation, and fatigue will vary. These factors obviously affect your training performance. Autoregulating your training allows you to go harder on days you're feeling powerful and motivated and pull back a bit when you're tired and beat up. This versatility amplifies your training effectiveness.

Auto-regulation uses a Rate of Perceived Exertion (RPE) scale for assessing each training set. The RPE rating quantifies, as objectively as possible, the difficulty of a given set. The System specifies a minimum and maximum RPE target for each set. These RPEs are listed in the training templates, and program structure descriptions. Appendix E describes the RPE scale. Examples of RPE ratings are:

RPE 10: You're at failure, you could not have done another rep (or you failed a planned rep).

RPE 8: This is a working weight, you still had two reps in the tank at the end of the set.

RPE 6: A relatively light set. Typically, a warm-up weight, or light accessory set.

Although rating the RPE of a given set remains somewhat subjective, don't overthink it. Give your best estimate based on how many reps you feel you had in the tank at the end of the set, bar speed, and how fatigued you are after completing the set. You'll find you get more accurate with RPE estimation with experience.

- RTS Emerging Strategies: Emerging Strategies is a training framework developed by Reactive Training Systems and has developed some of the strongest powerlifters in the world (as demonstrated by the number of RTS athletes competing at the IPF World Championships annually). The Emerging Strategies concept uses flexible programming, which allows you to react to emerging information about training performance and make necessary adjustments to maximize strengths and improve weaknesses. Although the System is built on a structured set of templates and tools, it is heavily influenced by the adaptability of Emerging Strategies.

  ○ Use of Estimated 1 Rep Max (e1RM): Each week's training is based off your current e1RM, not a fixed percentage of past maxes or future goals. Basing your training on your current e1RM sets your training intensity to what your strength level is now. Your e1RM sets the starting point for your weekly training. You may then adjust the actual training weight if necessary, through auto-regulation.

    I include tools you can use to calculate your e1RM on your primary lifts each week, and to calculate your planned weights. These tools will be discussed in Appendix F.

  ○ RPE/Intensity Reference Chart: I have adopted an RTS chart, which I include in Appendix E, that provides a target training percentage for a given RPE rating and repetition range. Use this chart and the tools listed above to calculate your weekly e1RMs and in planning your training weights.

○ Variable block length: True periodization plans, and most strength training programs, use fixed training block lengths. This simplifies training planning, but it results in less effective training. Because of the Law of Individual Differences discussed in chapter 1, athletes do not all peak at the same time. The time it takes for a body to adapt to a given stimulus is different from athlete to athlete.

Because of this I use a somewhat flexible duration for the training blocks in the System. I've structured each of the strength and power blocks to last between three and six weeks. I do apply some fixed structure but allow variability which should contain the time it takes to peak for most athletes.

I discuss adaptation and when to end your current block and move to the next further below in the program structure description and in appendix A.

○ Block modification: Once the body adapts to a stimulus, to continue building strength, you need to modify the input. At the end of a block you should have adapted well to the training in your current block (peaked). The training in the next block must be different enough to spur continued growth and strengthening. As the blocks progress, training volume and intensity change. These changes mimic periodization programs.

In addition to periodized changes, accessory lifts will change as well. For each block you will also select different accessory lifts. The lifts you choose should always be in line with the training you need most. Align them to address any weaknesses you have identified during your end of block assessments and any issues that arise during training.

Note: Unless you encounter a significant issue that prevents you from completing your training as planned, complete each training week consistently as your block is designed. Strength training is a skill. Give your body time to master the training in each block before you move to the next. Changing the training stimulus too frequently will dampen the effectiveness of this approach.

Program Structure

- Training Blocks: As alluded to in the paragraphs above, training is broken into a series of five training blocks. These blocks are described in detail in Appendix A. Each block consists of four training sessions that make up one training week, or microcycle. Appendix A describes the content of the training blocks, and Appendix B discusses the templates used to plan and document your actual training.

  The blocks that make up this program are:

  ○ Assessment Blocks: There is an assessment block at the beginning and end of the program (Blocks 1 and 5). Both are one week long and the purpose, as the name implies, is to assess your current training status. Block 1 assesses your strength level at the beginning of the program and establishes your key e1RMs. These will be used to plan subsequent training.

  ○ Strength Blocks: I define Blocks 2 and 3 as strength blocks. The intensity and volume used in these blocks are designed to build strength. These blocks vary in length between three and six weeks.

    When to end a strength or power block: You should continue using the current block to build your strength and skill until your body begins to adapt to the block's stimuli. Once you have adapted, you may find your performance, and e1RMs begin to drop. If your e1RMs drop for two consecutive weeks, you should move to the next block.

  ○ Power Block: I define Block 4 as the program's power block. Following basic periodization structure, the block's volume decreases and intensity increases. You'll find that reps per set decrease with subsequent blocks and the training percentages increase. The RPE ranges also increase slightly in Block 4. As a result, the target effect is an increase in power.

    For the purpose of this system:

    Strength is the general ability to generate force. It describes how many plates you can move on the bar.

Power is the ability to produce force quickly. Power relates to how explosively you can move a lot of plates on the bar.

- Training Sessions: As described above, each block is subdivided into four training sessions. The four sessions together make up a micro-cycle, or training week. The four training sessions are:

  Lower Body Push: The lower body push training session is your traditional 'leg day'. It is anchored by the squat and it emphasizes the quad heavily.

  Upper Body Push: Upper body push training is your 'bench day'. Bench Press is the primary lift for the session and it also trains in the vertical push plane with overhead presses.

  Lower Body Pull: Lower body pull training works your posterior chain (glutes, hamstrings and lower back). The primary lower body pull movement is the deadlift.

  Upper Body Pull: Upper body pull training works the upper back. Upper back training such as pull-ups and rows often get over-looked or glossed over with some low volume assistance work. A strong upper back is crucial in all heavy strength training, and it deserves as much emphasis as your bench training.

  Each of these four training sessions has the following general structure:

  Primary Lift: Each training session begins with a heavy compound lift that is the anchor to the target movement (squat, bench press, deadlift, barbell row). This is where the bulk of the training effect occurs.

  Assistance Lift: The assistance lift is also a compound lift with a similar pattern to the primary lift. In your lower body sessions, I like to use an assistance lift from the alternate movement pattern in this training slot. For instance, in the lower body push session, the assistance lift is a deadlift movement from the lower body pull pattern.

  Supplemental Lifts(s): Supplemental lifts are non-specific to the primary movement (the movement pattern is different; for instance, the close grip bench press is a specific movement pattern, as it mimics the bench press closely, whereas dips or dumbbell presses are less specific to the barbell bench press).

These lifts enhance the movement pattern and are most effective when they are selected to address weak areas in the primary movement pattern.

With this training system, I have specified which lifts will be used in the primary and assistance training slots. You will select supplemental lifts from the lift catalog. Pick lifts that you prefer based on a strength dimension you'd like to emphasize or a weakness you have identified during the assessment, as well as your personal preferences.

My goal with this session structure is to develop well balanced, full body strength.

- Training Volume Variability: I've included some variability in the overall volume for the System. Some of the lifts and sets have been flagged as optional in the templates. By including all possible lifts and sets you can complete the 'high' volume version of the program. The 'low' volume version leaves them out. Using the plan as listed without adding the optional lifts and sets results in the 'medium' version of the program.

Block 4 - Power

Lift Category	Lift	Volume and Intensity
Primary Squat	Back Squat	5 x 3 @ RPE 7.5-9 Start at 80% of E1RM Adjust to stay within RPE Range Volume Adjustments: High Volume: 6 x 3 Low Volume: 4 x 3

Figure 2-1 – Volume Variability

I have not programmed de-loads into the System. The purpose of variable volume is to allow you to bring the volume down in the event you begin to feel overtrained. It is best that you do not vary the volume frequently week to week, instead make these adjustments as you change blocks if possible. If modification is necessary mid-block, just make the minimum adjustment necessary in response to a specific cue, such as heavy fatigue.

Tools and Templates: Finally, I've included a set of tools which help you plan your training. Here is a brief introduction, but these tools and templates are described in detail in the appendices.

RPE Charts: Assigning an RPE number to a lift is a subjective task. I have, however, included charts to help add objectivity to the RPE assessment.

RPE Intensity Reference Chart: This is a reference that assigns a training percentage to a specific RPE at a target rep range. This is useful in determining a starting weight for a training session and is used to calculate your current e1RM.

Planned Weight and e1RM Calculators: Who wants to do the math? I've created spreadsheet formulas that will spit out your e1RM or planned starting weight for a given set once you plug in the appropriate information.

Lift Catalog: I've included a catalog of lifts I commonly use in my programming. You can use this catalog to pick out which supplemental lifts you'd like to use in your program.

Lift Weaknesses: Appendix D addresses common weaknesses in the squat, bench press, and deadlift, it provides recommendations (both technique and training) to address these limitations.

Training Log Templates: To accompany this book, I've built spreadsheet templates for each training session. You can use these templates to plan your sessions, log them during your training, and maintain a master training log of all your lifts. Logging your training is one of the most important aspects to effective training.

Assessment Log: At the end of each training block, document your results in the assessment log. It will help track your progress and spotlight areas that need emphasis.

Metrics Log: Track the weekly progress of your primary lifts using the metrics log. You will log your results here and document your weekly e1RMs for key lifts.

As you can tell by now, I use templates and tools associated with this program heavily. Much of this book is a reference to use these templates and tools effectively.

Now let's dig into each of the concepts for the System in more detail.

Chapter 3

KEY CONCEPTS: WARMING UP FOR TRAINING

Why is Warming Up Important?
Have you ever really thought about warming up or do you just get to work once you hit the gym? Warm-ups have some very important functions in preparing you to train.

- Prepares your body: A proper warmup elevates your heart rate and begins to pump more blood to your muscles. It increases your body temperature and the temperature of your muscles.
- Improves Mobility: Using your warmups for dynamic stretching loosens muscles acting on the target joint improving the range of motion and mobility around that joint.
- Primes your central nervous system (CNS): Using the proper weight selection as you warm up prepares the CNS to handle your training loads and tunes you up for the target lifting pattern.
- Reduces chances of injury: By raising your temperature, warming the muscles, improving mobility in the affected joints, and training your CNS for the target lifting patterns you reduce the chance of injury such as muscle pulls or strains.

An effective warmup strategy will make your training sessions more effective.

Should I stretch?

Optimally, your warm-ups will provide dynamic stretching you need. Use them to establish the mobility you need to complete your lifts with proper technique through the entire range of motion. As you do your assessment block and throughout your training, assess whether your mobility allows you to perform your lifts with proper technique and body positioning. If you identify mobility issues, focus your pre-lift mobility work in these areas.

If you do need additional stretching to improve mobility, add the stretches you need to develop that mobility. Save any static stretching until after you've performed enough warm-ups to bring your body and muscle temperature up a bit.

Mobility and pain: There are certain areas I have found where poor mobility leads to pain, both during and outside your training. Some simple mobility drills for these problem areas can have a surprisingly significant effect.

Note: These comments assume there is not an injury to these affected areas. Stretching will not improve an injury and you should consult a proper medical authority for proper treatment of all injuries and suspected injuries.

- Lower Back: I find that often lower back pain is caused by tight glute muscles tugging at your hip structure. This pain is localized in the lower back on one side or the other and is a dull throbbing pain (a sharp pain is an indication of an injury and should be addressed medically). Often, foam rolling the entire glute while consciously trying to relax the muscles can have a positive impact on this type of lower back pain. Roll the entire glute and pay special attention to the gluteus medius.
- Knees: Tight quads tend to pull on the patella, causing pain in the knee as you squat. Again, foam rolling can help address this pain. Foam roll the entire quad, particularly the painful outer sweep. Dynamic stretching, using lifts such as Bulgarian split squats, can also restore mobility to the quad and knee and is my go-to warm-up for squats before getting under the bar.
- Shoulders: Your shoulder is a relatively vulnerable joint. It provides movement in all planes of motion plus rotation. It is used to some

degree in all your lifts. It has a relatively shallow socket joint, whereas the hip sock is much deeper, making it much more vulnerable than the hip. It is important to maintain good mobility in the shoulder joint as well as strengthening the smaller muscles of the rotator cuff using light weights. Maintain flexibility in the pec muscles as well as the delts and lats to maintain shoulder mobility.

An extensive discussion on mobility is beyond the scope of this book. If you would like a very good and detailed tome addressing mobility for lifters, I highly recommend the book *Becoming a Supple Leopard* by Dr. Kelly Starrett. It discusses in detail how to address pain points caused by mobility issues.

What does my CNS do, and how does warming up affect it?
An important aspect of warming up is priming your CNS to lift heavy things. What exactly does the CNS do, you ask? The central nervous system is how the brain tells the muscles to move. Just like your muscular system, your CNS must also be trained to lift heavy weight.

This is a topic I find very interesting, but for the purpose of this book there are a couple key things to keep in mind.

- Your CNS becomes more efficient at engaging your musculature as you train. This neural efficiency allows you to engage more musculature more quickly and leads to greater strength production at the same level of muscle mass.
- The lifting pattern becomes more ingrained and natural as you train your CNS for it. You may find your lifting technique is a little rough as you start your warmups and gets cleaner as your warm-ups progress. By the time you get to your working sets you should be nailing it.

To illustrate my point, here is an example of my squat progression last night. The working sets were 5 x 5 at the same weight. I use the RPE scale to demonstrate the level of difficulty.

- Set 1: RPE 8.5
- Set 2: RPE 8
- Set 3: RPE 8

- Set 4: RPE 8
- Set 5: RPE 8.5

As you can see, my first set was tougher than sets 3-4, then set 5 again got tougher as fatigue set in. Even after warming up, my technique wasn't dialed in until my second working set, after which my body and CNS were well prepared for the training weight.

When thinking about warming up your CNS, it is important that your last warm-up set is heavy enough to get the body and CNS ready for the training weight, without inducing fatigue. As I state in the rules below, prepare the CNS by warming-up to within 5-10% of your working weight and using about half the reps you will use for training (if your working sets are singles, this does *NOT* mean you can half rep your warmups!).

In addition to getting your CNS firing efficiently, it is often useful to include some drills that will help activate the target muscle groups. These activation drills should be done before you start your lift specific warm-ups. Some examples might be:

- Glute activation drills prior to lower body training, such as glute bridges or Bulgarian split squats.
- Scapula activation drills prior to upper body training, such as face pulls or scapula pushups.

Warmup Rules

- Perform any non-specific warm-ups (mobility and muscle activation drills) before your lift specific warm-ups.
- Start with little or even no weight on the bar. Although light, consciously complete these warmup reps with perfect form to be sure you have the needed mobility for the target lifting pattern. For example, make sure you can squat to depth while maintaining good form.
- Target 4-6 sets of warm-ups. Don't use warm-ups to supplement your training volume, the weights used to warm-up are typically too low to create a useful training effect.
- Keep your reps per warm-up set lower than your training rep range. You may start with more reps at very light weights, but the bulk of

your warm-ups should be about half the number of reps of your working sets. Your warm-ups should not introduce fatigue before you get to your working sets.

- Use larger jumps in weight at the beginning of your warm-ups smaller jumps as you get closer to your training weight.
  Work up to within 5-10% of your starting weight.
- Approach every warm-up set with the deliberateness you give your heaviest working set. Consciously complete every warm-up rep with perfect technique.
- Since warm-up sets are lower intensity and volume, treat them as speed sets. Once you have developed your mobility through the full range of motion and have the muscles warm, complete the concentric portions of your warm-up reps with maximum speed and explosiveness.

Once you're warmed up, you should not be pre-fatigued and you should be ready to perform your working sets with proper technique throughout the lift's full range of motion. It's go time!

Chapter 4

KEY CONCEPTS: RPE AND AUTOREGULATION

"It doesn't matter how heavy it feels"

What does RPE stand for?
RPE stands for the Rate of Perceived Exertion. In simple terms, it measures the difficulty of your training.

You can find the standard RPE chart adopted from Reactive Training Systems in Appendix E. The scale varies from RPE 5.5 (easiest) to RPE 10 (most difficult) in .5 increments. At the low end of the scale RPE 5.5 is a very light warm-up requiring little real effort. There is no need to go lower on the scale than this.

RPE 10, at the upper end of the scale, represents a max effort set. If you hit failure (you are unable to complete all your reps or the set took every bit of strength and endurance you had), then an RPE 10 rating is appropriate.

How do I accurately determine what RPE to assign?
Between a failure set and the low end of the scale, the RPEs decrement based on how many reps you have left in the tank and your likelihood of hitting them.

- RPE 9.5: You *may* have had one rep in the tank

- RPE 9: You *definitely* had one rep in the tank

When assigning an RPE to a set, be as objective as you can, but don't overthink it. For effective training, consistency is more important than assignments scientifically measured to 99.999% accuracy. For instance, if you're not sure if the set was an RPE 8 or 8.5, and you're generally optimistic with your assessments, stick with the lower number. If you're generally conservative, select the higher number.

When assessing your RPE rating, there are several things to consider.

- How heavy does the weight feel: Use this measurement cautiously – it is a consideration, but it is the least reliable measurement of difficulty (my motto: It doesn't matter how heavy it feels).
- Bar speed: Does the bar speed move at your normal tempo? Faster? Slower?
- Technique: Was your technique off for the set? If so, was your technique off because of the bar weight, or did the bar weight seem heavier because your technique was off?

Based on these factors, could you have sucked it up and done another rep? Two more reps?

Note that you should be gauging these factors against a typical training session, not some absolute scale. Also keep in mind that this gauge may change over time as you become more seasoned.

How do I use RPEs in my training?
To discuss how to use your RPE assessment in training, we first need to understand autoregulation. Autoregulation is the concept of basing your training intensity on your level of preparedness in any given training session. Some days you just feel stronger. Maybe you're well rested, maybe you had a higher carb load in the previous few days. Whatever the case, on that given day you can lift heavier weights for more reps.

On the other hand, some days you feel like warmed up dung beetle excrement. Maybe you've been training hard without a break for a rest day and are feeling beaten down. Maybe you've just had a hard week at work and haven't been sleeping well. Whatever the case, you're more concerned with surviving your training than hitting PRs.

If you were following a static programming such as periodization, you won't have an optimal training session in either of these cases. Your plan will say seventy percent of last cycle's 1RM x 5 sets x 5 reps regardless of whether that weight is far too light or it crushes you.

With the System's autoregulation, on the other hand, you have a planned minimum and planned maximum RPE for each set. If you're feeling strong and completing your sets at or below the minimum RPE, you can bump the weight up. If the RPEs meet or exceed the maximum planned RPE, bring the weight down so you can complete all your assigned sets and reps.

I do have rules dictating when to adjust the weight.

1. When your RPE exceeds the maximum on your first set but you complete all the planned reps, try to complete two sets before lowering the weight. You'll find that at times it takes a set at your working weight to get your CNS and technique really dialed in.
2. If the weight is at or below the minimum RPE rating, complete at least three sets before raising the weight. Make sure you will be able to complete all your sets and reps in your latter sets as fatigue sets in.
3. If the weight is at or below the minimum RPE rating, but it will be progressing higher with each set, follow the plan, don't leapfrog planned weight increases.
4. When adjusting the weight up or down, start with around five percent changes in weight.

Note: These rules apply to the primary lifts for a session; adjust as necessary for accessory work.

Using RPE assignments and autoregulation you can squeeze the most out of your workouts. You lift more on strong days, less on weak days, but still hit your target training volume and intensity. This approach results in much more effective strength training.

Chapter 5

KEY CONCEPTS: YOUR 1RM AND e1RM

Everyone knows what a 1 rep max (1RM) is, but what is e1RM?
Okay, if you didn't know that 1RM stands for one rep max, you do now. Your 1RM is the most weight you have successfully completed in a specific lift at some point in time. It is your max. Your e1RM on the other hand, is your *estimated 1 rep max*. Your 1RM is how much you *have lifted*, e1RM quantifies how much you *can lift*.

Why is this distinction important? A couple reasons.

First, unless you were at failure the last time you maxed out, your 1RM isn't necessarily the most weight you could have lifted. Hitting a perfect 10 RPE while maxing out is incredibly unlikely. If you take big jumps in weight you may fail an attempt even if the previous set was easy – your true max is somewhere in between. If you take many smaller jumps you may fatigue early and hit failure while still below your true capability. Your 1RM represents how much you did lift; not how much you can lift. Your e1RM represents a better estimate of how much you are capable of lifting based both on how much you actually lifted, and how difficult the lift was.

Secondly, your 1RM represents how much you lifted at a point in time, and that time may have been many weeks or months ago. Your e1RM represents how much you can lift now (or more precisely, the last time you performed the target lift, which should be at most the previous week). Everyone experiences ups and downs in training. Your training plan should be flexible and allow adjustment for both the downs and the ups to make your training as effective as possible.

How do I find my e1RM?

Can't you just plug the weight and reps from your last set into one of those online one rep max calculators and have it spit out a number? Typical one rep max calculators miss a crucial variable in the equation – how difficult the set was. Properly assessing your e1RM considers the weight, number of reps, AND level of difficulty of the set.

Which set should you use to measure your e1RM? This is an important consideration. Some guidelines I use to select the set used for your e1RM measurement are:

- Select the set that used the highest weight.
- At that weight, pick the set with the most reps.
- With the given weight and reps, use the set with the lowest RPE rating.

Following these parameters, you will identify your strongest set for the microcycle. Basing your e1RM on this set should give you the best estimate of your current max.

Appendix F describes in detail how to use the estimated 1RM calculator I've included with the System's tools. Plug the numbers from the above training set and a percentage you find in the RPE/Intensity reference (Appendix E) into the e1RM calculator. This calculates your e1RM giving you a good indication of your current potential for a specific lift.

Keep in mind, although your e1RM should be a relatively close representation of your capability, it is an estimate. There are some factors that affects its accuracy.

- Sets with lower reps are typically more accurate than higher rep sets. More reps increase the subjectivity of your RPE assessment. Higher rep sets also introduce greater variability, introducing factors such as muscular fatigue and endurance levels. These factors complicate measuring strength levels.

- Higher RPE ratings are less subjective than lower RPE ratings (it's easier to tell if you have one rep in the tank versus three reps). These more objective and accurate RPE ratings increase the accuracy of your e1RM calculation.
- Your experience judging RPE ratings affects accuracy. As you train you gain a better understanding of each set's difficulty and how close to failure you are. As discussed, the more accurately you can estimate the RPE of a set, the closer to reality your e1RM will be.

How do I use the e1RM?

As I mentioned at the start of this chapter, basing your training on your e1RM versus some past 1RM helps you plan your training on your current strength level. It is not based on where you were at some point in the past, nor some arbitrary training goal. For the purpose of the System the e1RM has two functions.

- Use your e1RM to plan your training weights. To plan a session, plug the e1RMs from the previous week's training into the planned weight calculator (discussed in Appendix F). Use the calculated weight as the starting point for your training. You may then adjust, if necessary, to keep the actual intensity between the planned minimum and maximum RPEs listed in the training plan.
- Tracking your e1RM helps you track your progress. In addition to logging your training each week, I strongly recommend you record each week's e1RMs in the metrics log (Appendix I). This allows you to measure your progress weekly. You should notice that improving your technique and power at a given weight will demonstrate strength gains even if the weight on the bar remains the same. As you get more proficient with a lift, your RPE rating will come down at a given weight, which increases your e1RM. Technical proficiency and bar speed are nearly as important as is the actual bar weight.

The e1RM concept is fundamental to the System.

Chapter 6

KEY CONCEPTS: TRAINING ADAPTATION

*"Exercise is basically hurting yourself until you build up
an immunity to hurting yourself"* - Team Strength and Speed

How does lifting make me stronger?

Your body is an incredibly resilient mechanism. It has a tremendous capability to fight off disease and malady, heal itself, and adapt to its environment. Take your skin for example. Exposure to the sun causes it to tan (unless you're a redhead, sorry guys), protecting you from further burning.

Similarly, your body adapts to physical stimulus, preparing you better for the next exposure to it. The first time you try to squat three plates the weight may crush you. The second time you succeed, albeit with a bit of help from your spotter. The third time you kill the weight.

While this may be a dramatic oversimplification (the first time I tried to squat 650lbs, the weight crushed me and it took years after that to successfully lift 650lbs), your body does adapt to strength training by getting stronger. How does that happen?

There are many adaptations your body goes through when you start lifting. Here are some of the key changes that make you stronger.

- Increased muscle mass, aka hypertrophy: Simply put, as you lift weights your muscles get bigger. A top factor in determining muscular strength is the muscle's cross-sectional area. As your muscles get bigger, you get stronger.
- Greater tendon strength: As your muscles grow and become stronger and the weights you lift get heavier, your tendons also adapt. They grow stronger as well and capable of handling increasingly heavier loads. If this did not occur your joints would be unable to support the weight your muscles begin to move.
- Increased Central Nervous System (CNS) efficiency: Lifting heavy weights is as much a skill as it is an ability. To lift with peak effectiveness, you need the right muscles kicking on at the right times in the lift. As you practice lifting heavy weights, your CNS becomes more effective at firing the right muscles at the right times. It also increases in the ability to fire more muscle fibers more quickly. This is demonstrated both with greater technical skill and the ability to effectively move greater weights.

  Your CNS, as a protective mechanism, also tends to limit how much weight you lift. It does this to protect your body from injury (muscles, joints, tendons, etc.). When you first start lifting, your CNS does not understand how much you can safely lift and will shut you down if it perceives that the resistance too great. You can see this when a new lifter often fails suddenly, dropping without first slowing or stalling. An experienced lifter, on the other hand, has a much greater ability to grind at the weight, failure typically occurs less unexpectedly.
- Increased quantity of fast twitch muscle fibers: Although there is debate on whether an existing muscle fiber is capable of changing types, with strength training some amount of slow twitch muscle fibers begin to take on characteristics of fast twitch muscle fibers. This results in greater levels of explosive strength.

  Note: Fast twitch muscle fibers present characteristics of strength and power; slow twitch muscle fibers present characteristics of endurance.
- Maximizing energy systems for power: Strength training increases your body's ability to store higher levels of short-term energy sources (ATP, CP, creatine, glycogen).

Will these adaptations continue indefinitely?

I'm sure you've seen them. The people who do the same exact workout in the gym literally for years. They never seem to change or progress. Their bodies don't change. The weights they lift don't change.

While that may work for them, if you want to progress you have to challenge your body, give it a reason to adapt.

- Progressive Overload: Increasing your training weights will force your body to adapt and become stronger, for a time. At some point you will peak. Your strength will stop growing from simply adding more weight to the bar, it may even decline. At that point if you want to continue gaining strength, you need to modify other variables in your training as described later in the chapter.
- Law of Individual Differences: As I stated in chapter 1, every person is different. This applies to training adaptations as well; every person has their own time it takes to peak. Many training programs try to fit everyone into a tidy little box. While the programs may be effective and you may progress, adding flexibility to the program's duration and matching it to your individual time to peak can greatly increase its effectiveness.

How do I know when to change, and what do I change?

Although it is natural to have training ups and downs, the general trend of your training should be upward. A single downward week in the weight you lift in one or more of your three primary lifts (squat, bench press, deadlift) does not by itself indicate you have peaked. Instead look for downward trends in all three lifts (or multiple lifts) for consecutive weeks. When that happens, it is time to proceed to the next block.

In my experience, for experienced lifters the time to peak often falls between four to six weeks. If you are a new lifter (less than two years lifting experience), it is possible that you may progress much longer than six weeks. For the purpose of the System, however, at six weeks you will move on to the next training block even if your performance has not declined. The program changes the next block brings should spur even greater adaptations.

For the System, what changes in each block?

Following a block periodization model, volume and intensity will change in each subsequent training block (not including the assessment blocks at the beginning and end of the program).

- Volume: As each block progresses, training volume in the primary lifts as well as in the accessory lifts decreases. You will find that these lifts have fewer repetitions in each successive training block.
- Intensity: By virtue of the repetitions decreasing and given the same RPE range, you should have a corresponding increase in the weights you use. For your primary lifts, the starting percentages also increase and in the final power block the RPE range also increases slightly. I designed this system so that you continually challenge your body with heavier loads.

Although the primary lifts and key accessory lifts remain unchanged throughout the program, some lifts change from block to block. In each block you will select different accessory lifts.

- It is important that you do change these accessories versus using the same lifts throughout the entire program. These changes alter your program's stimulus and spur greater training adaptations.
- At the end of each block you will consciously assess where the weak points are in your lifts and your technique. Use this information to select accessory lifts and address and strengthen your weak points.

As you should be starting to see, I have designed the System to coax your body to adapt to training as effectively as possible for increased strength.

Chapter 7

KEY CONCEPTS: FATIGUE AND RECOVERY

"In bed is where the magic happens"

What is Fatigue?

I know what you're thinking, 'Fatigue? Fatigue is pretty self-explanatory, it's the reason I take afternoon naps before grabbing a pre-workout and heading off to the gym!' Maybe, but let's take a look under the covers. Let's discuss fatigue in the context of your training. In this sense, I am referring to the reduction in your ability to create the powerful muscular contractions necessary to move big weights. As fatigue builds, your ability to create force deteriorates and in extreme cases, ceases.

I'd like to differentiate between the fatigue that occurs between sets during your training, recovering between your training sessions, and discuss overtraining briefly.

During your training

During a training session, accumulation of fatigue limits how many reps you can complete within a set at a given weight. Although the central nervous system (CNS) can be a factor (see the discussion below), an important limiter for an individual set's intensity and volume is the depletion of energy stores. There are two primary energy stores used during anaerobic activity.

- Adenosine triphosphate (ATP): ATP provides immediate energy for explosive movements. At maximum effort ATP is depleted very quickly – in a matter of seconds. Once depleted, your body shifts to the second energy source, the glycolytic pathway. ATP stores are typically restored in a few minutes.
- Glycolytic Pathway: Once you've burned through your ATP stores, your body breaks down glycogen within the body to create more ATP. The glycolytic pathway can sustain one to two minutes of heavy training. Although you won't deplete this energy store to the point you cannot generate energy, your body begins to build up waste within the muscles more rapidly than you can flush them out introducing fatigue (and pain) and limiting your set.

Your rest periods should be such that you can replenish energy stores, flush out waste products, and continue lifting at the target training intensity. Typically, you are ready to resume training within three to five minutes or less, depending on your training volume and intensity and your conditioning level.

Between training sessions, you need to give your body time to recover from the damage caused by your heavy training.

- Heavy training creates micro-tears in your muscle fibers. This is normal and one of the factors that causes muscle soreness post training. It also is a stimulus prompting your body to rebuild itself stronger than before. It is natural. You do, however, need to give your body time to recover from the damage your training has inflicted.
- Generating energy also causes accumulation of by-products within the muscle cells. This waste is not completely flushed during your training session.

Typically, your body can recover from a training session within forty-eight to seventy-two hours. It is advisable to avoid training the same muscular systems on consecutive days to allow for recovery. If you do train the same system within that window, the subsequent session should be at a lower intensity. You must also monitor your recovery over time to be sure that fatigue is not accumulating week to week. There are several factors that can affect how quickly you recover from your training session. To get the best training results, pay attention to what you're doing outside the gym as well.

- Training Volume: Understand that high volume training takes longer to recover from. Take that into account when you schedule your training split.
- Sleep: Sleep is vital to your recovery. It allows your body to repair itself and reduces levels of stress induced hormones such as cortisol. Everyone is different, of course, but if you're training heavy, at least eight hours of good, uninterrupted sleep is a good target.
- Stress: We all have many stressors outside the gym in everyday life. Life stress (work, family, emotional state, etc.) compounds the physical stress your training demands. Addressing external stress and striving for a balanced lifestyle aids your ability to recover. Periods of high external stress, such as a demanding work schedule, may require you to scale back your training volume.
- Hydration: Drink your water. It's been said that if you are dehydrated to the point that you feel thirsty, your physical performance can be affected significantly. Losing even two percent of your body's water mass can cause a two to three percent decrease in strength and power performance.
- Conditioning: Cardio gets a bad rap in the strength and power circles. However, maintaining good physical conditioning can help you recover faster, train harder, and get stronger. Your conditioning should favor intensity over duration. Long periods of steady state cardio, such as thirty minutes on a treadmill, does not translate as well for heavy strength training as shorter more intense sessions.
- Age: Keep in mind that as you age, your recovery may take longer. Consistent training and conditioning will help but pay attention to the indicators that you need more recovery time and adjust if you need to.

What role does my CNS play in recovery?
Your CNS is responsible for your voluntary muscular contractions. When you are preforming any movement, squatting for example, you want your brain to

tell your legs to bend. You send this message from your brain through your CNS to the muscles in your legs, glutes, hamstrings, quads (and pretty much everything else in the case of squats) telling them to contract or relax (so they can stretch).

The CNS can also act as a governor. It deliberately limits your power output if it detects the potential for injury. It does this by limiting the contractile force you are able to produce in your muscles. As you train with heavy weights your CNS becomes more efficient at signaling strong contractions and allowing you to train with greater power. However, when the CNS starts to detect fatigue conditions, and/or potential injuries (pain), it begins to limit that power.

Recovery is more complex than simply sucking it up and doing the work. Which brings me to my final point, overtraining.

How can I tell if I am over-trained, and what should I do?
Let's begin with an understanding of what overtraining is. Simply being sore from your last training session *does not* mean you are overtrained. It *does not* excuse you from today's squat session. Overtraining occurs when your training volume exceeds your body's ability to recover from that training over time. If this lack of recovery occurs over an extended period, fatigue builds up and begins affecting your performance. Some symptoms of overtraining include:

- Lack of energy
- Achy joints
- Decreased lifting performance
- General lack of motivation
- Increased incidents of injury, or generally more injury prone

Muscle soreness from training is not in and of itself an indication of overtraining. Soreness is normal, particularly during periods where activity levels or specific movements have changed significantly. Although you may need more time to warm up and prepare to lift, muscle soreness should not affect your training significantly.

Since overtraining can result when your training volume exceeds your body's ability to recover, there are two approaches to addressing overtraining: increase your body's ability to recover or reduce your training volume.

How can I improve my body's ability to recover?

-   Make sure you are getting adequate sleep. As discussed above, sleep is crucial to your training recovery. Properly recovering prevents overtraining.
-   Feed the machine. As with sleep, diet is an important aspect to your recovery. Consuming adequate carbohydrates replenishes fuel needed for energy, and protein provides the building blocks necessary to repair damaged muscle fibers.
-   Reduce training induced inflammation. Take care of your body. Two of the best methods to reduce inflammation and aid recovery are getting a massage and cool (ice) water immersion.

Let's say you have healthy eating and sleeping habits. What's next, how do you go about reducing your training volume? The training templates with the System provides you with options for high, normal and low volume.

-   If you have a high training capacity, you may decide to add the optional sets and lifts associated with a high volume approach. These optional high volume sets and reps are indicated in the program block descriptions (Appendix A), and the training templates (Appendix B). If you feel you are not recovering adequately as the program progresses, stop adding these sets and lifts to your sessions.
-   To complete the normal volume, complete the lifts in the templates as designed, without adding high volume sets and lifts.
-   To drop to the low volume approach, reduce the number of sets as listed in the templates and block descriptions for low volume.
-   If you are using the low volume approach and you are still exhibiting symptoms of overtraining, you may need to take more aggressive and drastic action. You can reduce training volume further by eliminating the last supplemental lift in each training session. Keep in mind that this could affect the balance of your training, and your effectiveness in addressing weaknesses.

Taking care to ensure you are recovering can be as important to your results as your actual lifting.

Appendix A

PROGRAM STRUCTURE – THE TRAINING PLAN

The overall program described by this system may appear daunting and complex at first, but let's break it down into its component parts. The individual components are more easily digestible. When addressing a complex problem, I like to start with the big picture, and drill down in detail until everything comes together.

The System is not a workout template, it is a training system. It is broken down into a series of blocks, micro-cycles (training weeks), and training sessions. Through this appendix I will describe each block and training session in detail.

Block 1 - Assessment		Block 2 - Strength		Block 3 - Strength		Block 4 - Power		Block 5 - Assessment	
Purpose	Duration	Purpose	Duration	Purpose	Duration	Purpose	Duration	Purpose	Duration
Asess Primary Lifts	1 Week	Build Strength	3-6 Weeks	Build Strength	3-6 Weeks	Build Power	3-6 Weeks	Assess Program Results	1 Week

Figure A-1: Program Blocks

I discuss the program block structure briefly in Chapter 2, Training Approach. I'll cover it here in much greater detail.

Block 1 – Assessment:
Before you begin training, you need to know a couple things:

- What are you capable of lifting?
- What are your weaknesses?

The purpose of the assessment block is to answer these questions. This block is one week long and has relatively low volume. I'll describe the specific block content later in this appendix, but the intent of this block, as mentioned, is to determine the starting point for your program, you're not building strength…yet.

Blocks 2 and 3 – Strength Building:
Blocks 2 and 3 are designed to build a solid, well balanced foundation in strength. The volume and intensity are set in a range to maximize strength gains and the lift selection addresses all the major muscular systems with a relative balance.

These two blocks are a minimum of three weeks and a maximum of six weeks long. By completing at least three weeks in a block, you build skill with the selected lifts at an intensity to maximize strength gains. After completing three weeks, if you have two consecutive weeks with a decline in the e1RMs of the primary lifts (squat, bench press, deadlift), then that block should be ended. This approach is designed to allow you to build as much strength in each block as possible and moving on to the next block once you've peaked. If you have not experienced any declines after six weeks, end the block and move to the next one anyway. The metrics log in Appendix I will help you track when it is appropriate to end the current block and proceed to the next one.

As the blocks progress, using the periodization approach, the program's volume will decrease, and the intensity will increase.

Block 4 – Power:
Through the normal periodized progression, when you reach Block 4, the program's intensity and volume will be optimized to build the power attribute of your strength. The volume will be lower than previous blocks, and the intensity will be higher. The System also increases the RPE range for this block to the range I prefer for power sessions.

As with Blocks 2 and 3, the duration of this block will be a minimum of three weeks and a maximum of six weeks. Also, as with previous blocks, if you have two consecutive weeks of declining e1RMs, end the block, and move to the final assessment block.

Block 5 – Assessment:

The structure of Block 5 is largely the same as Block 1. Block 5 is also one week in length and relatively low volume. The intent of this block is to re-assess your lifts and determine how much strength you have gained based on your new e1RMs. If the program has progressed well, you should set new actual 3RMs as well.

You should also take this time to assess the program's impact on your weaknesses. Have they been resolved? Have new weaknesses been uncovered?

Why are three rep sets and e1RMs used to measure progress instead of working up to a 1RM? The System, as the name implies, is designed to build strength for beginners. Using 3RMs versus 1RMs keeps the weight a bit lighter, reducing the injury risk. It is my preference to use 1RMs only for intermediate to advanced lifters with very sound lifting technique.

Now that you have the big picture, let's see what the blocks look like.

Block 1 - Assessment			
Training Session	Lift Category	Lift	Volume and Intensity
Session 1 - Squat Assessment	Primary Squat	Back Squat	5 Sets 1 x 3 @ RPE 8 85% of your 1RM if known Work up to 3 Reps @ RPE 9 If less than 5 sets, drop back to RPE 8 and finish sets
	Squat Accessory	Lower Body Push supplemental lift	3 x 10 @ RPE 6.5-8

Figure A-2: Block 1 – Session 1 – Squat Assessment

Session Structure:

All training sessions in all program blocks are set up with a consistent structure. The first session of the first training block is displayed above in figure A-2.

- *Training Session*: The first column in this table lists the name of the training session. There are four training sessions in each block and the name should give a good indication of the training goals for that session. The four training sessions will make up your training week, or microcycle.
- *Lift Category*: The lift category identifies what type of lift will be performed in that training slot. The first training slot is used for your primary lift for that day. In figure A-2, since this is a squat assessment, this slot is used for your primary squat. Subsequent training slots are used for lifts that support your primary lift. In this figure slot two is

used for a squat accessory lift.

- *Lift*: The lift column names the specific lift you will perform in the training session. For the Squat Assessment session this will be the back squat. You'll notice slot two does not name a specific lift, instead lists 'Lower Body Push supplemental lift'. In this case you will select a lift from the catalog (or your favorite supplemental lift) that corresponds to this type of lift.

- *Volume and Intensity*: The final column describes the volume, in sets and reps, and the weights to use.
  - ○ Volume is listed in sets x reps format.
  - ○ Intensity will be listed either in a percentage of your e1RM or by a target minimum and maximum RPE.
    - If the weight is planned correctly, for your early sets you should remain in the low end of the RPE range, and as fatigue builds your latter sets will creep up closer to the maximum end of the RPE range.
    - Don't adjust the weight up too quickly if the weight feels light. Unless the weight is below the minimum RPE, complete at least three sets before increasing the weight.

For the best results using this system, you should plan your training sessions in advance, including any optional lifts and specific target weights to use. I've included training templates you can use to document your plan (Appendix B). You can easily use these templates to plan and document your training.

Note that warmups and any mobility work are not listed in the program structure. For each session make sure you include adequate mobility and warmup sets and exercises before getting into the listed working sets.

One final word before we dive in. You will have ups and downs through the course of this program, as you will with any training program. Trust the process and work through the low points. Take advantage of the high points and concentrate on long term progress. Use the flexibility this program provides to make course corrections you require, but don't hop to something new at the first sign of a challenge.

Block 1 – Assessment

The purpose of the Block 1 is to determine your strength level and identify weaknesses to be addressed. As with all other blocks in the System, it consists of four training sessions.

Session 1 – Squat Assessment:
During session one, you will assess your relative strength level in the back squat and perform some limited accessory work.

- Slot 1 – Primary Squat: The first lift you will perform is the back squat. You will perform a total of five sets. If you have a recent, known 1RM, set your first working set to eighty-five percent of that weight, after your mobilization and warmups. If you are unsure of your current 1RM, work up to an RPE 8 during your warm-ups and use that as your first working set. Increase the weight in each subsequent set until you reach an RPE rating of 9. For any remaining sets drop back to a weight you can complete at an RPE 8 difficulty.
- Slot 2 – Squat Accessory: In the second slot perform an assistance lift for the back squat. The program allows you to select an accessory of your choice. In the lift catalog, you will find lifts with the category lower body push, supplemental for this training slot. You may also choose other lifts you prefer, if they fall into the lower body push category. For your squat accessory lift you will perform three sets of ten reps between the RPEs of 6.5 (minimum) and 8 (maximum).

During Block 1, there are relatively few lifts you will perform. The intent is not to work to failure, but to identify your strengths and weaknesses, and prepare you for the strength work starting in Block 2.

Session 2 – Bench Press Assessment:

Block 1 - Assessment			
Training Session	Lift Category	Lift	Volume and Intensity
Session 2 - Bench Press Assessment	Primary Bench Press	Bench Press	5 Sets 1 x 3 @ RPE 8 85% of your 1RM if known Work up to 3 Reps @ RPE 9 If less than 5 sets, drop back to RPE 8 and finish sets
	Bench Press Accessory	Upper Body Push supplemental lift	3 x 10 @ RPE 6.5-8
	Primary Shoulder	Standing Overhead Press	1 x 5 @ RPE 8 Work up to 5 reps @ RPE 9

Figure A-3: Block 1 – Session 2 – Bench Press Assessment

The purpose of session two is to assess your strength level in the bench press. Session two also includes the standing overhead press for shoulder strength development and some limited bench press accessory work. Throughout this system, shoulder training will be incorporated into your bench press sessions since they are both considered pushing movements for the upper body.

- Slot 1 – Primary Bench Press: The approach to assessing your bench press is like your squat assessment. You will perform a total of five sets. The first set starts at eighty-five percent of your 1RM, if known, after your mobilization and warmups. As with squats, if you are unsure of your current 1RM, work up to an RPE 8 during your warm-ups, and use that as your first working set. Increase the weight in each subsequent set until you reach an RPE rating of 9. For any remaining sets drop back to a weight you can complete at an RPE 8 difficulty.
- Slot 2 – Bench Press Accessory: The second slot in this session is a supplemental lift for the bench press. Select the accessory you prefer to support your bench press from the lift catalog with the category upper body push, supplemental. Again, you may choose other lifts you prefer, if they fall into this category. For your bench press accessory, you will complete three sets of ten reps between RPEs 6.5 and 8.
- Slot 3 – Primary Shoulder: Throughout this program, the standing overhead press will be used as your primary shoulder lift. You will perform sets of five reps, starting at RPE 8, and working up to an RPE of 9.

As with your squat assessment session, the intent of this session is not to train excessively hard. The purpose is to gauge where you are at in the bench press and overhead press so you may plan future sessions appropriately.

Session 3 – Deadlift Assessment:

Block 1 - Assessment			
Training Session	Lift Category	Lift	Volume and Intensity
Session 3 - Deadlift Assessment	Primary Deadlift	Sumo or Conventional Deadlift	5 Sets 1 x 3 @ RPE 7 75% of your 1RM if known Work up to 3 Reps @ RPE 8
	Deadlift Accessory	Lower Body Pull supplemental lift	3 x 10 @ RPE 6.5-8

Figure A-4: Block 1 – Session 3 – Deadlift Assessment

During session three you will assess your deadlift strength. Session three addresses the strength in your posterior chain (glutes, hamstrings, lower back) and accessory work for posterior chain strength development.

-   Slot 1 – Primary Deadlift: For your primary deadlift you may use either the conventional deadlift or sumo deadlift. Use the deadlift style you are most comfortable with, stronger at, and can use the best technique with. If you are unsure, use both approaches during the assessment, alternating styles for each set. When you've finished this session, you should be able to select as a primary deadlift the form you performed the best.

    For the assessment you will perform a total of five sets. If you are testing both conventional and sumo deadlifts, complete six sets, performing both deadlift styles at each weight. Since deadlifts are more taxing on the body, your intensity will be lower. Start at seventy-five percent of your 1RM, or a weight you can complete with RPE 7. Increase the weight for each set and work up to an RPE 8. If there are any remaining sets, drop back to an RPE 7 to complete them.

    If you are testing both sumo and conventional and the RPE ratings are different between them, base the RPE rating for the assessment on the style with the lower RPE. For example, if the RPE for sumo is 7.5 and for conventional it is 8, continue increasing the weight for the next sets until you hit RPE 8 with the sumo deadlift as well. In this example, if you consistently rate sumo deadlifts with a lower RPE (and both have equally good technique), you should consider sumo deadlifts as your primary form.

- Slot 2 – Deadlift Accessory: Select the accessory you prefer to support your deadlift and train your posterior chain. You may pick a lift from the catalog with the category lower body pull, supplemental, or choose other lifts you prefer of this type. For the deadlift accessory, you will complete three sets of ten reps between RPEs 6.5 and 8.

Session 4 – Back Assessment:

Block 1 - Assessment			
Training Session	Lift Category	Lift	Volume and Intensity
Session 4 - Back Assessments	Back - Horizontal	Barbell Rows	5 Sets 1 x 5 @ RPE 7 Work up to 5 reps @ RPE 8.5
	Back - Vertical	Pull-ups	3 x AMRAP
	Upper Back Accessory	Upper Body Pull supplemental lift	3 x 10 @ RPE 8-9.5

Figure A-5: Block 1 – Session 4 – Back Assessment

Session four, your back assessment, is a bit different from other sessions in Block 1 for a couple reasons.

- For balance, the back should be trained in two planes: horizontal and vertical. This is accomplished by including both rows (horizontal) and pull-ups (vertical) in your back training sessions.
- I don't use 1RMs for back training because max effort rows can be problematic. They put a lot of torque on the lower back, and it is nearly impossible to complete near max weight with strict form. I've also found the upper back responds better to high volume using a moderate weight than it does to low volume with near max weights.

For these reasons, rows and pull-ups are used throughout this training system with lower weight and higher volume than lifts in other training sessions.

- Slot 1 – Back – Horizontal/Rows: Barbell rows are performed first. Training horizontal rows harder, with more volume and intensity translates to greater back support for the big three lifts – squats, bench press and deadlifts.

    For the purpose of the System, select weights for barbell rows that you can perform with strict form, use little or no upper body momentum to assist the lift.

You will do a total of five sets of five reps. Start with a weight, after warming up, that you can complete all five reps at RPE 7. Work up to a weight that you can complete your reps at RPE 8.5 and finish your sets at that weight. If you need to use body momentum to cheat and get all your reps, reduce the weight for subsequent sets.

- Slot 2 – Back – Vertical/Pull-ups: Pull-ups are, without a doubt, the best vertical pulling lift there is. For this session, and throughout the System, you will perform all your sets for an AMRAP (As Many Reps as Possible). If you are unable to get at least five reps (don't feel bad, you're not alone), use assistance for them. You can do this by using a resistance band or an assisted pull-up machine.
- Slot 3 – Upper Back Accessory: You will perform three sets of ten reps of an upper back accessory lift of your choosing. Select a lift from the lift catalog or you may pick your own personal favorite. It should be an upper body pull supplemental lift.

As you complete each session, document the results in your training log. Appendix B discusses how to use the System templates to plan and document your training. As you complete each session, you should also capture key information that will help you measure progress and plan future sessions:

- Logging metrics is described in Appendix I.
- Measuring your e1RM is discussed in Appendix F.
- Use Appendix H to address weaknesses and identify technical issues you may have with your lifts.

Taking the few moments required to jot down this information will make your training much more productive.

Block 2 – Strength

After completing Block 1 you should have a good idea where your strength levels lie and what your e1RMs are for your primary lifts. You should have also identified weaknesses and technique issues you need to address. This information will help plan your training as you progress.

Block 2 is designed to begin building a solid, well balanced foundation in strength. It accomplishes this through the design of the volume, intensity, and selection of lifts. This block and the remaining building blocks, are set up with an upper/lower, push/pull structure:

- Session 1: Lower Body Push
- Session 2: Upper Body Push
- Session 3: Lower Body Pull
- Session 4: Upper Body Pull

Using this design, and laying out your training week, there are a couple things you should keep in mind:

- Alternate upper body and lower body training sessions as shown to allow for maximum recovery time for similar muscular and energy systems.
- When possible, schedule your training week to prevent more than two rest days between training sessions.

The structure of the sessions in Block 2 is like the assessment block, albeit with heightened intensity and volume.

As discussed in Block 1, it is important to keep records of your training so you that may track your progress and properly plan future training sessions as each block progresses. You will also use these records to identify when you have peaked and should move on to the next block.

Session 1 – Lower Push:
The primary purpose of this training session is to build your squat strength. As you will note, it also includes deadlift assistance work.

Block 2 - Strength 1			
Training Session	Lift Category	Lift	Volume and Intensity
Session 1 - Lower Push	Primary Squat	Back Squat	5 x 5 @ RPE 7-8.5 Start at 75% of E1RM Adjust to stay within RPE Range Volume Adjustments: High Volume: 6 x 5 Low Volume: 4 x 5
	Deadlift Assistance	Speed Deadlifts Alternate Deadlift Type	4 x 3 @ RPE 6-7.5 Start at 60% of your deadlift E1RM Volume Adjstments: High Volume: 6 x 3
	Squat Supplemental	Lower Body Push supplemental lift	3 x 10 @ RPE 6.5-8
	High Volume	Add Lower Body Push isolation lift	3 x 12 @ RPE 8-9.5

Figure A-6: Block 2 – Session 1 – Lower Push

First, a bit of housekeeping, since there are some new concepts in this session which were not present in your assessment block.

- Use of e1RM: You calculated your e1RM as you completed your assessment block and hopefully recorded it in your metrics log. This is an important concept. Basing your training on your most current e1RM allows you to adjust your training intensity based on your most current strength level assessment.
- Volume Adjustments: I believe training volume is a key factor in building strength and durability. For this reason, the System is built with moderately high training volume. However, every lifter is a bit different with respect to their response to training volume. I have therefor included some flexibility in the training volume. Due to the balanced nature of this system, I do recommend sticking to the program as designed, and the pre-defined adjustments. Adding additional lifts and volume won't necessarily improve your performance over the course of the program. I do also recommend performing the base program for at least one to two weeks before adjusting, provided you are recovering adequately between training sessions.

There are four training slots in this training session, with the fourth one being optional for a higher volume training session.

- Slot 1 – Primary Squat: Perform five sets of five reps, starting at seventy-five percent of the e1RM you set the previous week. Adjust the weight if necessary, to stay above the minimum RPE 7 and below the maximum RPE 8.5.
  - To use the high-volume approach, complete six sets.
  - To use the low-volume approach, complete only four sets.
- Slot 2 – Deadlift Assistance: Perform speed deadlifts using the alternate deadlift approach. If your primary deadlift is conventional, these will be done sumo and vice versa. Complete four sets of three, starting at sixty percent of your deadlift e1RM set the previous week (this is the e1RM of your *primary deadlift*). These should be light, explosive lifts with perfect technique. The RPE should remain low and bar speed high for all sets, between RPE 6 – 7.5.

- For the high-volume approach, complete six sets.
- Slot 3 – Squat Supplemental: Select a supplemental lift for the lower body push movement. You may select a lift from the lift catalog, or one of your own choosing. This should not be an isolation movement (single joint movement, such as leg extensions). You may substitute a lower body push assistance lift but be aware that these are generally quite similar to the primary movement, and more taxing than most supplemental lifts. Choose a lift that directly impacts any weaknesses or technique issues you discover during your lift assessments.

    Note: As a personal preference, I really like using leg press or hack squat in this training slot.

    You will use the same supplemental lift throughout this training block, then change it for subsequent blocks.
- Slot 4 – Lower Body Isolation – Optional/High Volume: You may add this lift to add volume to your squat session. It should be a low impact, single joint isolation movement such as the leg extension. As with your supplemental lifts, use this training slot to address weaknesses in your squats.

Complete three sets of twelve reps between RPE 8 – 9.5.

Record your results and prepare for session 2!

Session 2 – Upper Push:
It's Bench Day, everyone's favorite!

Block 2 - Strength 1			
Training Session	Lift Category	Lift	Volume and Intensity
Session 2 - Upper Push	Primary Bench Press	Bench Press	5 x 5 @ RPE 7-8.5 Start at 75% of E1RM Adjust to stay within RPE Range Volume Adjustments: High Volume: 6 x 5 Low Volume: 4 x 5
	Bench Press Supplemental	Upper Body Push Supplemental Lift	3 x 10 @ RPE 6.5-8
	Primary Shoulder	Standing Overhead Press	3 x 10 @ RPE 6.5-8
	High Volume	Add Upper Body Push isolation lift	3 x 15 @ RPE 8-9.5

Figure A-7: Block 2 – Session 2 – Upper Push

The structure for your bench session is like the squat session you just completed.

- Slot 1 – Primary Bench Press: Perform five sets of five reps, starting at seventy-five percent of the e1RM you set the previous week. Adjust the weight if necessary, to stay above the minimum RPE 7 and below the maximum RPE 8.5.
  - To use the high-volume approach, complete six sets.
  - To use the low-volume approach, complete four sets.
- Slot 2 – Bench Press Supplemental: Select a supplemental lift for the upper body push movement. You may select a lift from the lift catalog, or one of your own choosing. Select a lift that will directly impact any bench press weaknesses or technique issues you discover during your assessment. You will use the same supplemental lift throughout this training block.

  If you are using the lift catalog, you may want to substitute an assistance lift versus a supplemental lift, depending on your training goals.

  Complete three sets of ten reps between RPE 6.5 – 8.
- Slot 3 – Primary Shoulder: As discussed in Block 1, you will use the Standing Overhead Press to strengthen your shoulders throughout this program. Complete 3 sets of 10 reps between RPE 6.5 – 8. As the shoulder is a vulnerable joint, keep this weight on the low end of the RPE range, using weights you can complete with perfect technique.
- Slot 4 – Upper Body Isolation – Optional/High Volume: You may add this lift to add volume to your bench press session. It should be a single joint isolation movement, such as triceps extensions or pec flyes. As with your supplemental lifts, use this training slot to address weaknesses in your bench press. Given this movement is lower impact, the repetition and RPE range will be higher.

Complete three sets of fifteen reps between RPE 8 – 9.5.

Record your results, let's get ready to pull!

Session 3 – Lower Pull:

Session 3 is your deadlift session. Deadlifts are one of the most taxing lifts, for this reason I limit the high volume adjustments in the System.

Block 2 - Strength 1			
Training Session	Lift Category	Lift	Volume and Intensity
Session 3 - Lower Pull	Primary Deadlift	Conventional or Sumo Deadlift	5 x 5 @ RPE 6.5-8 Start at 65% of E1RM Adjust to stay within RPE Range Volume Adjustments: Low Volume: 4 x 5
	Squat Assistance	Lower Body Push assistance lift	3 x 8 @ RPE 6.5-8
	Deadlift Supplemental	Lower Body Pull supplemental Lift	3 x 10 @ RPE 6.5-8
	High Volume	Add Lower Body Pull isolation lift	3 x 15 @ RPE 8-9.5

Figure A-8: Block 2 – Session 3 – Lower Pull

This session is somewhat of a mirror image to your squat session. Your primary lift is the deadlift and it is supplemented with a squat movement.

- Slot 1 – Primary Deadlift: Your primary deadlift is the deadlift style you found to be stronger and better technique during your assessment, either conventional or sumo. You will use this same deadlift style throughout this program. It is possible that you'll find at the end of the program the other style has become stronger or easier to perform with good form. During the program, however, you should remain consistent with one style.

    Perform five sets of five reps, starting at sixty-five percent of the e1RM you set the previous week. Adjust the weight if necessary, to stay between RPEs 6.5 – 8. Because of the toll deadlifts take on the entire body, I reduce the intensity for them slightly.
    - To use the low-volume approach, complete only four sets.
    - There is no high-volume deadlift adjustment.
- Slot 2 – Squat Assistance: You will perform a squat assistance lift on deadlift day. It should be squat-specific movement pattern, although less specific, supplemental movements such as front squats and Zercher squats are also acceptable. The lift you use should not be the same as used during your squat session. Keep the weight relatively light for this lift and focus closely on maintaining perfect technique.

Complete three sets of eight reps for your squat assistance between RPE 6.5 – 8.

- Slot 3 – Deadlift Supplemental: As with all supplemental lifts, select an exercise that will strengthen any areas of weakness and technique flaws. For this training session, it needs to isolate the posterior chain (glutes, hamstrings, lower back).

    Perform three sets of ten reps at RPE 6.5 – 8.

- Slot 4 – Lower Body Isolation – Optional/High Volume: You may add this lift to add volume to your deadlift session. It should be a single joint, low impact isolation movement, such as leg curls or kettlebell swings. Use this slot to add volume if you need it, and to address weak areas in your deadlift.

Complete three sets of fifteen reps between RPE 8 – 9.5.

One more session for this week, but it's a biggie – the back!

Session 4 – Upper Pull:
Session 4, the final session in each week of Block 2, is your upper back training. Because of the important role your back plays in every one of your big lifts, it deserves its own training session.

Block 2 - Strength 1			
Training Session	Lift Category	Lift	Volume and Intensity
Session 4 - Upper Pull	Upper Body Pull, Primary	Barbell Rows	5 x 6 @ RPE 7-8.5
	Upper Body Pull, Assistance	Pull-Ups	3 x AMRAP Use assistance or added weight if necessary - target is 6-10 reps
	Upper Body Pull, Supplemental	Upper Body Pull Assistance / Supplemental Lift	3 x 15 @ RPE 8-9.5
	High Volume	Add Upper Body Pull isolation lift	3 x 15 @ RPE 8-9.5

Figure A-9: Block 2 – Session 4 – Upper Pull

As with the back assessment session, this session centers around pulling movements in both the vertical (pull-ups) plane, and horizontal (rowing) plane.

- Slot 1 – Upper Body Pull, Primary: For the duration of this program, the primary upper back movement is the barbell row. When executed properly, barbell rows are a very effective strength building tool for your back!

Perform five sets of six reps at an RPE between 7 – 8.5.

You won't measure e1RMs for barbell rows. When selecting your starting weights, review the weight used and RPE measurements from your previous week. Adjust the weight as necessary to stay within the RPE boundaries. For the purpose of this program, complete your barbell rows with strict form, using minimal body movement for assistance.

- Slot 2 – Upper Body Pull, Assistance: Pull-ups will be used throughout the System for the vertical upper body pulling movement. If you are unable to get at least six reps on your own, use assistance (resistance bands or an assisted pull-up machine). If you can complete ten reps unassisted you may want to add some additional weight. Try to reduce assistance and/or increase additional weight as the program proceeds.

  Complete three sets of as many reps as possible; target is at least six full range of motion reps.

- Slot 3 – Upper Body Pull, Supplemental: Select a supplemental lift from the lift catalog or one of your choosing. You may also substitute upper body pull assistance lifts into this slot if you prefer. My preference is to use a horizontal/rowing accessory movement in this slot, versus a vertical pulling movement.

  Complete three sets of fifteen reps with RPE ranging between 8 – 9.5.

- Slot 4 – Upper Body Isolation – Optional/High Volume: If you want to add additional volume to the upper body pull session, you may include this training slot in your session. It should be a low impact isolation movement. Although rowing and pulling movements do work the biceps, this is a good training slot to plug in some form of bicep curls.

As I emphasize throughout this program, document the results for each training session. For the best results capture your lifts as you go, or shortly after your session. Note any improvements in weak movements and new problem areas you discover. You will use this information from week to week to plan upcoming training sessions. After week three of the block, review your training metrics as discussed in Appendix I to determine when it is appropriate to end Block 2 and move on to Block 3.

Block 3 – Strength

Block 3 is also a strength block and the overall structure mimics Block 2 closely. Volume in your primary lifts is reduced slightly and intensity is increased. The target for this block is to increase the weight 2-5% above the weight you used in Block 2 – provided you stay within the RPE constraints. The primary intent is to continue building on the strength you developed in Block 2.

Because Block 3 looks much like Block 2, in this section I will emphasize the differences.

Session 1 – Lower Push:

Block 3 - Strength 2			
Training Session	Lift Category	Lift	Volume and Intensity
Session 1 - Lower Push	Primary Squat	Back Squat	5 x 4 @ RPE 7-8.5 Start at 77% of E1RM Adjust to stay within RPE Range Volume Adjustments: High Volume: 6 x 4 Low Volume: 4 x 4
	Deadlift Assistance	Speed Deadlifts Alternate Deadlift Type	4 x 3 @ RPE 6-7.5 Start at 65% of your deadlift E1RM Volume Adjstments: High Volume: 6 x 3
	Squat Supplemental	Lower Body Push supplemental lift Select different lift than previous block	3 x 8 @ RPE 6.5-8
	High Volume	Add Lower Body Push isolation lift	3 x 12 @ RPE 8-9.5

Figure A-10: Block 3 – Session 1 – Lower Push

You will have the same number of training slots in this block as in Block 2. Except for the squat supplemental slot, the lifts will remain the same. You will select a different exercise for slot 3 to change this block's training stimulus.

- Slot 1 – Primary Squat: Perform five sets of four reps, starting at seventy-seven percent of your current e1RM. Adjust the weight needed to stay above the minimum RPE 7 and below the maximum RPE 8.5.
  - To use the high-volume approach, complete six sets.
  - To use the low-volume approach, complete four sets.

  For this block the number of reps drops from five to four and the starting weight increased to seventy-seven percent of your E1RM.

Your RPEs remain the same.

- Slot 2 – Deadlift Assistance: Perform speed deadlifts using your alternate deadlift approach. Complete four sets of three, starting at sixty-five percent of your deadlift e1RM set the previous week. Keep RPEs low for all sets, between RPE 6 – 7.5. Focus on lifting explosively with perfect technique. Try and make every rep faster than the previous rep, and every set faster than the previous set.
  - For the high-volume approach, complete six sets.
- Slot 3 – Squat Supplemental: Select a new supplemental lift for the lower body push movement. You may select a lift from the lift catalog, or one of your own choosing. Choose a different supplemental lift than you used in Block 2, you will use this lift throughout Block 3.

  Choose a lift that will directly address weaknesses or technique issues you discovered during your lift assessment, or any new issues that have emerged during Block 2.

  Perform three sets of eight reps between RPE 6.5-8.

  Note: The more different this exercise is from Block 2's supplemental lift the better. For example, if you feel you need to work your quad strength and you used leg presses in Block 2, maybe you want to try front squats or Zercher squats in Block 3.
- Slot 4 – Lower Body Isolation – Optional/High Volume: You may add this lift to add volume to your squat session. It should be a single joint isolation movement. As with your supplemental lifts, use this training slot to address weaknesses in your squats. If you used slot 4 in Block 2, select a different lift for this block if you can.

  Complete three sets of twelve reps between RPE 8 – 9.5.

Record your results and press on.

Session 2 – Upper Push:

Block 3 - Strength 2			
Training Session	Lift Category	Lift	Volume and Intensity
Session 2 - Upper Push	Primary Bench Press	Bench Press	5 x 4 @ RPE 7-8.5 Start at 77% of E1RM Adjust to stay within RPE Range Volume Adjustments: High Volume: 6 x 4 Low Volume: 4 x 4
	Bench Press Supplemental	Upper Body Push Supplemental Lift Select different lift than previous block	3 x 8 @ RPE 6.5-8
	Primary Shoulder	Standing Overhead Press	3 x 8 @ RPE 6.5-8
	High Volume	Add Upper Body Push isolation lift	3 x 15 @ RPE 8-9.5

Figure A-11: Block 3 – Session 2 – Upper Push

As with session 1, your bench press session looks very much like Block 2, except the reps go down slightly and the weight will go up.

- Slot 1 – Primary Bench Press: Perform five sets of four reps, starting at seventy-seven percent of your current e1RM. Your RPEs stay between the minimum RPE 7 and maximum RPE 8.5.
    - To use the high-volume approach, complete six sets.
    - To use the low-volume approach, complete four sets.
- Slot 2 – Bench Press Supplemental: Select a new supplemental lift for the upper body push movement. This should be different than the lift you used in Block 2. Identify a lift that will address any bench press weaknesses or technique issues you have identified. You will use the same supplemental lift throughout Block 3.

    Complete three sets of eight reps between RPE 6.5 – 8.
- Slot 3 – Primary Shoulder: The standing overhead press will remain your primary shoulder exercise. Complete three sets of eight reps between RPE 6.5 – 8. Keep the weight at a level you can complete all reps with perfect technique.
- Slot 4 – Upper Body Isolation – Optional/High Volume: Include this slot to add volume to your bench press session if desired. Use a single joint isolation movement and select a different lift than used in Block 2, if you used this slot. As with all supplemental lifts, use this training slot to address weaknesses in your bench press.

    Complete three sets of fifteen reps between RPE 8 – 9.5.

As always, record your lifts and chalk up for deadlifts!

Session 3 – Lower Pull:

Block 3 - Strength 2			
Training Session	Lift Category	Lift	Volume and Intensity
Session 3 - Lower Pull	Primary Deadlift	Conventional or Sumo Deadlift	5 x 4 @ RPE 6.5-8 Start at 70% of E1RM Adjust to stay within RPE Range Volume Adjustments: Low Volume: 4 x 4
	Squat Assistance	Lower Body Push assistance lift Use different lift than previous block	3 x 8 @ RPE 6.5-8
	Deadlift Supplemental	Lower Body Pull supplemental Lift Select different lift than previous block	3 x 8 @ RPE 6.5-8
	High Volume	Add Lower Body Pull isolation lift	3 x 15 @ RPE 8-9.5

Figure A-12: Block 3 – Session 3 – Lower Pull

As with other sessions in Block 3, weight increases, and volume decreases for your deadlift session. Select different lifts for both the squat assistance and deadlift supplemental lifts.

- Slot 1 – Primary Deadlift: Use the same deadlift style (conventional or sumo) for your primary deadlift as you used in Block 2.
  Perform five sets of four reps, starting at seventy percent of your current deadlift e1RM. Keep your sets between RPEs 6.5 – 8.
  ○ To use the low-volume approach, complete four sets.
- Slot 2 – Squat Assistance: Select a new squat-specific movement pattern to use as an assistance lift. It should not be the same as the supplemental lift you used in your squat session or the squat assistance lift for Block 2. Keep the weight relatively light for this lift, focus on perfecting your technique.
  Complete three sets of eight reps for your squat assistance between RPE 6.5 – 8.
- Slot 3 – Deadlift Supplemental: Select a new supplemental lift for the posterior chain. Perform three sets of eight reps at RPE 6.5 – 8.
- Slot 4 – Lower Body Isolation – Optional/High Volume: You may add a lower body isolation lift, as in Block 2, to add volume to your deadlift session. It should be a single joint, low impact isolation movement, different from any used in Block 2.
  Complete three sets of fifteen reps between RPE 8 – 9.5.

Document your deadlift session and get ready for your last session in block 3.

Session 4 – Upper Pull:
Session 4 wraps up Block 3 training each week with upper back training.

Block 3 - Strength 2			
Training Session	Lift Category	Lift	Volume and Intensity
Session 4 - Upper Pull	Upper Body Pull, Primary	Barbell Rows	4 x 6 @ RPE 7-8.5 Volume Adjustment - for both High and Medium Volume add: 1 Drop Set - AMRAP at 10RM - AMRAP at -25% - AMRAP at -50%
	Upper Body Pull, Assistance	Pull-Ups	3 x AMRAP Use assistance or added weight if necessary - target 8-12 reps
	Upper Body Push Assistance	Speed Bench Press Use alternate Grip (wide, med, close) Short rest periods	4 x 3 @ RPE 6-7.5 Start at 65% of your deadlift E1RM Volume Adjustment: High Volume: 6 x 3
	Upper Body Pull, Supplemental	Upper Body Pull Assitance / Supplemental Lift Select different lift than previous block	3 x 15 @ RPE 8-9.5
	High Volume	Add Upper Body Pull isolation lift	3 x 15 @ RPE 8-9.5

Figure A-13: Block 3 – Session 4 – Upper Pull

Session 4 increases weight and decreases volume per set, as in other Block 3 sessions. This session also introduces a new approach, *drop sets* and adds bench press *speed sets*, as described below.

- Slot 1 – Upper Body Pull, Primary: Barbell rows, perform four sets of six reps at an RPE between 7 – 8.5 with strict form.
  - For both high and medium volume sessions, the fifth set will be a drop set: Begin with a 10RM weight and do as many reps as possible. Rack the bar and quickly strip off twenty-five percent of the weight and immediately continue your set with no rest, again completing as many reps as you can. Rack the weight and strip off another twenty-five percent and continue to failure a third time.

    If possible, set up your bar so you can quickly strip weight plates off. Don't add smaller plates to be more precise with the total bar weight. For example: start at 135lbs with a 25lb plate and two 10lb plates on each side. For each drop pull a 10lb weight off each side and continue.

    For best results, have training partners strip the weight down for each drop so you can continue with the exercise more quickly.

- For low-volume, complete only four sets with no drop set.
  - Slot 2 – Upper Body Pull, Assistance: Do three sets of pull-ups to failure. If you are unable to get at least eight reps on your own, use some form of assistance. If you can complete twelve reps unassisted, do them with additional weight.
  - Slot 3 – Upper Body Push, Assistance: Block 3 adds the speed bench press to improve your explosive power and tune your bench press technique. For speed sets use a normal speed eccentric and pause at the chest. *Blast* the bar off your chest as explosively as possible. Try to complete each repetition faster than the previous rep, and each set faster than the set before.

    Complete four sets of three reps with RPEs from 6-7.5. Start with sixty-five percent of your current bench press e1RM for your first set. The weight should remain relatively light, so that you can maintain explosive bar speed. Keep your rest periods for these sets relatively short as well. Complete each subsequent set as soon as you feel recovered, but no longer than two minutes.

    Note: use a different grip than you use in your primary bench press for the speed bench, either narrower or wider.
  - Slot 4 – Upper Body Pull, Supplemental: Select a new upper body pulling supplemental lift for Block 3. It should be a different exercise than used in Block 2 and should address weaknesses in you have identified.

    Complete three sets of fifteen reps with RPE ranging between 8 – 9.5.
  - Slot 4 – Upper Body Isolation – Optional/High Volume: To add additional volume to this session, you can include a low impact isolation movement.
    - If you include it, do three sets of fifteen reps with the RPE between 8 – 9.5.

Collect your results for each training session and at the end of each week update your training metrics as described in Appendix I. After week three of the block, review the metrics to determine when to move on to Block 4.

Block 4 – Power

Structurally, Block 4 looks very similar to blocks 2 and 3, you will complete four sessions each with three to five training slots. Block 4 again increases the intensity and reduces training volume into what I consider the *power range* (one to three reps for your primary lifts). As well as a higher bar weight and fewer reps in this block, I also increase the RPE range slightly in this block.

Since the System is targeted at novice lifters, you will not train with fewer than three reps.

This will be your final building block, and by this point in the program you should have built a firm strength foundation. Take advantage of that and push the edge a bit.

Session 1 – Lower Push:

Block 4 - Power			
Training Session	Lift Category	Lift	Volume and Intensity
Session 1 - Lower Push	Primary Squat	Back Squat	5 x 3 @ RPE 7.5-9 Start at 80% of E1RM Adjust to stay within RPE Range Volume Adjustments: High Volume: 6 x 3 Low Volume: 4 x 3
	Deadlift Assistance	Speed Deadlifts Alternate Deadlift Type	4 x 3 @ RPE 6-7.5 Start at 67% of your deadlift E1RM Volume Adjstments: High Volume: 6 x 3
	Squat Supplemental	Lower Body Push supplemental lift Select different lift than previous block	3 x 8 @ RPE 6.5-8
	High Volume	Add Lower Body Push isolation lift	3 x 12 @ RPE 8-9.5

Figure A-14: Block 4 – Session 1 – Lower Push

- Slot 1 – Primary Squat: Perform five sets of three reps, starting at eighty percent of your current e1RM. Adjust the weight needed to stay above the minimum RPE 7.5 and below the maximum RPE 9.
  - To use the high-volume approach, complete six sets.
  - To use the low-volume approach, complete four sets.

  For this block the number of reps drops from four to three, which should result in a higher weight for this block. You also start at a higher percentage of your e1RM for your first set, and your RPE range is slightly higher than previous blocks.
- Slot 2 – Deadlift Assistance: Perform speed deadlifts using your alternate deadlift approach. Complete four sets of three, starting at

sixty-seven percent of your deadlift e1RM set the previous week. Keep RPEs between RPE 6 – 7.5 and focus on the explosiveness of each rep. Maintain perfect technique and try to increase the bar speed with each rep, try to make every set faster than the previous set.

- ○ For the high-volume approach, complete six sets.
- Slot 3 – Squat Supplemental: Select a new supplemental lift for the lower body push movement. Choose a different supplemental lift than you used in blocks 2 and 3.

  Choose a lift that will directly address weaknesses or technique issues you discovered during your lift assessment and any new issues that have emerged during blocks 2 and 3.

  Perform three sets of eight reps between RPE 6.5-8.
- Slot 4 – Lower Body Isolation – Optional/High Volume: You may add a single joint isolation lift to add volume to your squat session. The lift you choose should be different than any you used in blocks 2 and 3.

  Complete three sets of twelve reps between RPE 8 – 9.5.

As always, finish your training session by recording your results (if you haven't recorded them between sets of your session).

Session 2 – Upper Push:

Block 4 - Power			
Training Session	Lift Category	Lift	Volume and Intensity
Session 2 - Upper Push	Primary Bench Press	Bench Press	5 x 3 @ RPE 7.5-9 Start at 80% of E1RM Adjust to stay within RPE Range Volume Adjustments: High Volume: 6 x 3 Low Volume: 4 x 3
	Bench Press Supplemental	Upper Body Push Supplemental Lift Select different lift than previous block	3 x 8 @ RPE 6.5-8
	Primary Shoulder	Standing Overhead Press	4 x 6 @ RPE 6.5-8
	High Volume	Add Upper Body Push isolation lift	3 x 15 @ RPE 8-9.5

Figure A-15: Block 4 – Session 2 – Upper Push

Your bench press session in Block 4 also has a higher training weight and lower volume.

- Slot 1 – Primary Bench Press: Perform five sets of three reps, starting at eighty percent of your current e1RM. Your RPEs increase to a minimum RPE 7.5 and maximum RPE 9.
  ○ To use the high-volume approach, complete six sets.
  ○ To use the low-volume approach, complete four sets.
- Slot 2 – Bench Press Supplemental: Select a supplemental lift for the upper body push movement that is different than the ones you used in blocks 2 and 3. Use this training slot to continue working on your weaknesses.

  Complete three sets of eight reps between RPE 6.5 – 8.
- Slot 3 – Primary Shoulder: The Standing Overhead Press will remain your primary shoulder exercise.

  Complete four sets of six reps between RPE 6.5 – 8. Keep the weight at a level you can complete all reps within the RPE range and with perfect technique.
- Slot 4 – Upper Body Isolation – Optional/High Volume: Include an upper body push isolation lift to add volume to your bench press session. Choose a different lift than used in blocks 2 and 3.

  Complete three sets of fifteen reps between RPE 8 – 9.5.

Update your training records so you are ready for the next session.

Session 3 – Lower Pull:

Block 4 - Power			
Training Session	Lift Category	Lift	Volume and Intensity
Session 3 - Lower Pull	Primary Deadlift	Conventional or Sumo Deadlift	5 x 3 @ RPE 7-8.5 Start at 75% of E1RM Adjust to stay within RPE Range Volume Adjustments: Low Volume: 4 x 3
	Squat Assistance	Lower Body Push assistance lift Use different lift than previous block	3 x 6 @ RPE 6.5-8
	Deadlift Supplemental	Lower Body Pull supplemental Lift Select different lift than previous block	3 x 8 @ RPE 6.5-8
	High Volume	Add Lower Body Pull isolation lift	3 x 15 @ RPE 8-9.5

Figure A-16: Block 4 – Session 3 – Lower Pull

The intensity will increase in session 3, as in earlier sessions. Again, because deadlifts are more taxing on the body, the CNS, and the soul, relative intensity for deadlifts will be kept slightly lower than for other lifts.

- Slot 1 – Primary Deadlift: Maintain the same primary deadlift style through the end of this last heavy block.

  Perform five sets of three reps, starting at seventy-five percent of your current deadlift e1RM. Keep your sets between RPE 7 – 8.5.
  ○ To use the low-volume approach, complete four sets.
- Slot 2 – Squat Assistance: Select a squat-specific assistance movement, different from the assistance lifts you used in blocks 2 and 3. You will use a moderate weight and need to maintain good lift technique.

  Complete three sets of six reps for your squat assistance between RPE 6.5 – 8.
- Slot 3 – Deadlift Supplemental: Select a new posterior chain supplemental lift.

  Perform three sets of eight reps at RPE 6.5 – 8.
- Slot 4 – Lower Body Isolation – Optional/High Volume: You may include a lower body isolation lift to add volume to your deadlift session. It should be a single joint, low impact isolation movement, different from any used in blocks 2 and 3.

  Complete three sets of fifteen reps between RPE 8 – 9.5.

Update your training log and move on to session 4.

Session 4 – Upper Pull:

Block 4 - Power			
Training Session	Lift Category	Lift	Volume and Intensity
Session 4 - Upper Pull	Upper Body Pull, Primary	Barbell Rows	4 x 6 @ RPE 7.5-9 Volume Adjustment - for High and Medium Volume add: 1 Drop Set - AMRAP at 8RM - AMRAP at -25% - AMRAP at -50%
	Upper Body Pull, Assistance	Pull-Ups	3 x AMRAP Use assistance or added weight if necessary - target 8-12 reps
	Upper Body Push Assistance	Speed Bench Press Use alternate Grip (wide, med, close) Short rest periods	4 x 3 @ RPE 6-7.5 Start at 70% of your deadlift E1RM Volume Adjustment: High Volume: 6 x 3
	Upper Body Pull, Supplemental	Upper Body Pull Assitance / Supplemental Lift Select different lift than previous block	3 x 15 @ RPE 8-9.5
	High Volume	Add Upper Body Pull isolation lift	3 x 15 @ RPE 8-9.5

Figure A-17: Block 4 – Session 4 – Upper Pull

For session 4 of this block the changes from Block 3 are more subtle than in other Block 4 training sessions. I call these changes out below.

- Slot 1 – Upper Body Pull, Primary: Barbell rows, perform four sets of six reps, as in Block 3. The RPE for this block increases to 7.5 – 9, again with strict form.

  The last set of barbell rows in this block remains a drop set (high and medium volume), but the starting weight increases from a 10RM to an 8RM. If you are unsure of the difference in weight between 10RM and 8RM, increase the weight around ten percent from your most recent upper body pull session.
  - Begin with an 8RM weight, perform as many reps as possible. Rack the bar and quickly strip off twenty-five percent of the weight continue your set with no rest, again working to failure. Rack the weight and strip off another twenty-five percent and continue to failure a third time. As described in Block 3, set up your bar so you can quickly strip weight plates off for each round.
  - For low-volume, complete only four sets with no drop set.
- Slot 2 – Upper Body Pull, Assistance: Perform three sets of pull-ups to failure. If you can't complete at least eight reps, use some form of assistance. If you can complete twelve or more reps unassisted, do them with additional weight.
- Slot 3 – Upper Body Push, Assistance: Continue using the Speed Bench Press to improve your explosive power and tune your bench press technique.

  Complete four sets of three reps with RPEs from 6-7.5. Start with seventy percent of your current bench press e1RM for your first set. Keep the weight light enough so that you maintain explosive bar speed for all your sets and reps. Keep your rest periods relatively short.

  For high volume, complete six sets of three reps.

  Use a different grip than you used in Block 3 for the speed bench (either wider or narrower).
- Slot 4 – Upper Body Pull, Supplemental: Select a different upper body pulling supplemental lift for Block 4. Choose an exercise that you haven't used previously.

  Complete three sets of fifteen reps with RPE ranging between 8 – 9.5.

- Slot 4 – Upper Body Isolation – Optional/High Volume: To add additional volume to this session, you can include a low impact isolation movement.

    Complete three sets of fifteen reps with the RPE between 8 – 9.5.

Document your training results for each session. Update your metrics at the end of each training week to determine when to end Block 4.

Block 5 – Assessment

By the time you reach Block 5, you have done a tremendous amount of work. The purpose of Block 5 is to measure the results of your hard work. Do keep in mind that progress is not always measured in lbs and kgs on the bar. In some cases, it can be measured in significant improvements in your technique.

The training sessions in Block 5 will mirror Block 1 very closely. The purpose is to measure improvement in your lifts between your first week and last week using this system.

The volume in this block will be relatively low. Although you will be testing your lifts with heavier weights, this block should also be used for recovery from any fatigue that has built up.

Session 1 – Squat Assessment:

Block 5 - Assessment			
Training Session	Lift Category	Lift	Volume and Intensity
Session 1 - Squat Assessment	Primary Squat	Back Squat	5 Sets 1 x 3 @ RPE 8 85% of your E1RM Work up to 3 Reps @ RPE 9 If less than 5 sets, drop back to RPE 8 and finish sets
	Squat Accessory	Lower Body Push supplemental lift	3 x 10 @ RPE 6.5-8

Figure A-18: Block 5 – Session 1 – Squat Assessment

As in Block 1 you will assess your relative strength level in the back squat. The volume for this session (and all of Block 5) will be relatively low, with limited accessory work.

- Slot 1 – Primary Squat: Start at eight-five percent of your current e1RM for a set of three reps and work up to a set with 9 RPE. Weight increases for each set should be between five to ten percent.

Complete a total of five sets of three reps. If you reach RPE 9 in less than five sets, drop your weight back to complete the rest of your sets at RPE 8.

- Slot 2 – Squat Accessory: Select a lower body push supplemental lift. As opposed to previous blocks, you can re-use an accessory lift in Block 5.
Perform three sets of ten reps at RPE 6.5 – 8.

As with all previous blocks, be sure to record each session's results.

Session 2 – Bench Press Assessment:

Block 5 - Assessment			
Training Session	Lift Category	Lift	Volume and Intensity
Session 2 - Bench Press Assessment	Primary Bench Press	Bench Press	5 Sets 1 x 3 @ RPE 8 85% of your E1RM Work up to 3 Reps @ RPE 9 If less than 5 sets, drop back to RPE 8 and finish sets
	Bench Press Accessory	Upper Body Push supplemental lift	3 x 10 @ RPE 6.5-8
	Primary Shoulder	Standing Overhead Press	1 x 5 @ RPE 8 80% of your E1RM Work up to 5 reps @ RPE 9

Figure A-19: Block 5 – Session 2 – Bench Press Assessment

Although the main purpose of this session to is to assess your bench press, you will also assess your vertical pressing strength with the overhead press.

- Slot 1 – Primary Bench Press: Retest your bench press strength. Start at eighty-five percent of your current e1RM and complete a set of three reps. Increase each subsequent set by five to ten percent until you reach RPE 9.
Complete a total of five sets of three reps. If you reach RPE 9 before finishing all five sets, drop the weight back and complete any remaining sets at RPE 8.
- Slot 2 – Bench Press Accessory: Select an upper body push supplemental lift. As with your squat session, it is okay in Block 5 if this is an accessory you have previously used.
Perform three sets of ten reps between RPEs 6.5 and 8.
- Slot 3 – Primary Shoulder: Test your overhead press strength. Start at eighty percent of your current overhead press e1RM and complete

a set of five reps. Increase the weight each set until you reach an RPE 9. Once you reach RPE 9, you are finished.

Session 3 – Deadlift Assessment:

Block 5 - Assessment			
Training Session	Lift Category	Lift	Volume and Intensity
Session 3 - Deadlift Assessment	Primary Deadlift	Sumo or Conventional Deadlift	5 Sets 1 x 3 @ RPE 7 75% of your E1RM Work up to 3 Reps @ RPE 8 If less than 5 sets, drop back to RPE 7 and finish sets
	Deadlift Accessory	Lower Body Pull supplemental lift	3 x 10 @ RPE 6.5-8

Figure A-20: Block 5 – Session 3 – Deadlift Assessment

During session 3, you will assess your deadlift progress.

- Slot 1 – Primary Deadlift: For the assessment, use the same primary deadlift style that you have used throughout the program. Start with seventy-five percent of your current deadlift e1RM for a set of three reps. Increase the weight by five to ten per set until you reach a set with an RPE of 8.

   Complete a total of five sets of three reps. If you have remaining sets after reaching RPE 8, drop back to RPE 7 to complete your sets.
- Slot 2 – Deadlift Accessory: Select a lower body pull exercise to perform as your accessory lift.

   Complete three sets of ten reps between RPEs 6.5 and 8.

Session 4 – Back Assessment:

Block 5 - Assessment			
Training Session	Lift Category	Lift	Volume and Intensity
Session 4 - Accessory Assessments	Back - Horizontal	Barbell Rows	5 Sets 1 x 5 @ RPE 7 Work up to 5 reps @ RPE 8.5 If less than 5 sets, drop back to RPE 7 and finish sets
	Back - Vertical	Pull-ups	3 x AMRAP
	Upper Back Accessory	Upper Body Pull supplemental lift	3 x 10 @ RPE 8-9.5

Figure A-21: Block 5 – Session 4 – Back Assessment

Session 4 will assess your back strength in both the horizontal and vertical planes.

- Slot 1 – Back – Horizontal/Rows: Start with a set of 5 reps at RPE 7. Increase the weight for each subsequent set five to ten percent until you reach RPE 8.5.

    You will complete a total of five sets of five reps. If you reach RPE 8.5 before completing all sets, drop back to RPE 7 to complete your remaining sets.

    All sets should be completed with strict form.
- Slot 2 – Back – Vertical/Pull-ups: For Block 5, if possible complete your pull-ups without assistance, and without additional weight. Complete three sets to failure.
- Slot 3 – Upper Back Accessory: Perform three sets of ten reps of an upper back accessory lift of your choice.

Wrapping up your training cycle:
At the end of Block 5, you should review your results for the entire program. Some things to look at are:

- What were your strength gains in each primary lift?
- How did your lifting technique improve?
- Did you see improvement in your weaknesses?
- Have new weaknesses or technique flaws been identified?

Documenting your results will help you plan your future training cycles. After completing this training cycle and assessment, you may want to run the cycle again, starting right in with Block 2 or move to a new program – but don't stop!

Training Session Shorthand:
For those of you who prefer a simple representation of the program, I've included a short hand description for each training block. This also is a handy reference to use once you understand the training system.

Block 1:

Block 1
Session 1 - Squat Assessment
Back Squats, 5 x 3
- Work up to RPE 9, then back off to RPE 8
Lower Body Push Supplemental, 3 x 10 @ RPE 6.5-8
Session 2 - Bench Press Assessment
Bench Press, 5 x 3
- Work up to RPE 9, then back off to RPE 8
Upper Body Push Supplemental, 3 x 10 @ RPE 6.5-8
Standing Overhead Press, 3 x 5
- Work up to RPE 9, then back off to RPE 8
Session 3 - Deadlift Assessment
Deadlift, Conventional, 5 x 3
- Work up to RPE 8, then back off to RPE 7
Lower Body Pull Supplemental, 3 x 10 @ RPE 6.5-8
Session 4 - Accessory Assessments
Barbell Rows, 5 x 5
- Work up to RPE 8.5, then back off to RPE 7
Pull-ups, 3 x AMRAP
Upper Body Pull Supplemental, 3 x 10 @ RPE 8-9.5

Figure A-22: Block 1 Shorthand

Block 2:

Block 2
Session 1 - Lower Body Push
Back Squats, 5 x 5 @ RPE 7-8.5
- Low Volume: 4 x 5
- High Volume: 6 x 5
Speed Deadlift, Sumo, 4 x 3 @ RPE 6-7.5
- High Volume, 6 x 3
Lower Body Push Supplemental, 3 x 10 @ RPE 6.5-8
Lower Body Push Isolation, 3 x 12 @ RPE 8-9.5
- High Volume only
Session 2 - Upper Body Push
Bench Press, 5 x 5 @ RPE 7-8.5
- Low Volume: 4 x 5
- High Volume: 6 x 5
Upper Body Push Supplemental, 3 x 10 @ RPE 6.5-8
Standing Overhead Press, 3 x 10 @ RPE 6.5-8
Upper Body Push Isolation, 3 x 15 @ RPE 8-9.5
- High Volume only
Session 3 - Lower Body Pull
Deadlift, Conventional, 5 x 5 @ RPE 6.5-8
- Low Volume: 4 x 5
Lower Body Push Assistance, 3 x 8 @ RPE 6.5-8
Lower Body Pull Supplemental, 3 x 10 @ RPE 6.5-8
Lower Body Pull Isolation, 3 x 15 @ RPE 8-9.5
- High Volume only
Session 4 - Upper Body Pull
Barbell Rows, 5 x 6 @ RPE 7-8.5
Pull-ups, 3 x AMRAP
Upper Body Pull Supplemental, 3 x 15 @ RPE 8-9.5
Upper Body Pull Isolation, 3 x 15 @ RPE 8-9.5
- High Volume only

Figure A-23: Block 2 Shorthand

Block 3:

Block 3
Session 1 - Lower Body Push
Back Squats, 5 x 4 @ RPE 7-8.5
- Low Volume: 4 x 4
- High Volume: 6 x 4
Speed Deadlift, Sumo, 4 x 3 @ RPE 6-7.5
- High Volume, 6 x 3
Lower Body Push Supplemental, 3 x 8 @ RPE 6.5-8
Lower Body Push Isolation, 3 x 12 @ RPE 8-9.5
- High Volume only
Session 2 - Upper Body Push
Bench Press, 5 x 4 @ RPE 7-8.5
- Low Volume: 4 x 4
- High Volume: 6 x 4
Upper Body Push Supplemental, 3 x 8 @ RPE 6.5-8
Standing Overhead Press, 3 x 8 @ RPE 6.5-8
Upper Body Push Isolation, 3 x 15 @ RPE 8-9.5
- High Volume only
Session 3 - Lower Body Pull
Deadlift, Conventional, 5 x 4 @ RPE 6.5-8
- Low Volume: 4 x 4
Lower Body Push Assistance, 3 x 8 @ RPE 6.5-8
Lower Body Pull Supplemental, 3 x 8 @ RPE 6.5-8
Lower Body Pull Isolation, 3 x 15 @ RPE 8-9.5
- High Volume only
Session 4 - Upper Body Pull
Barbell Rows, 4 x 6 @ RPE 7-8.5
Barbell Row Drop Set: 10RM, 10RM - 25%, 10RM - 50% for AMRAPs
- For High AND Medium Volume
Pull-ups, 3 x AMRAP
Speed Bench Press, 4 x 3 @ RPE 6-7.5
- High Volume: 6 x 3
Upper Body Pull Supplemental, 3 x 15 @ RPE 8-9.5
Upper Body Pull Isolation, 3 x 15 @ RPE 8-9.5
- High Volume only

Figure A-24: Block 3 Shorthand

Block 4:

Block 4
Session 1 - Lower Body Push
Back Squats, 5 x 3 @ RPE 7.5-9
- Low Volume: 4 x 3
- High Volume: 6 x 3
Speed Deadlift, Sumo, 4 x 3 @ RPE 6-7.5
- High Volume, 6 x 3
Lower Body Push Supplemental, 3 x 8 @ RPE 6.5-8
Lower Body Push Isolation, 3 x 12 @ RPE 8-9.5
- High Volume only
Session 2 - Upper Body Push
Bench Press, 5 x 3 @ RPE 7.5-9
- Low Volume: 4 x 3
- High Volume: 6 x 3
Upper Body Push Supplemental, 3 x 8 @ RPE 6.5-8
Standing Overhead Press, 4 x 6 @ RPE 6.5-8
Upper Body Push Isolation, 3 x 15 @ RPE 8-9.5
- High Volume only
Session 3 - Lower Body Pull
Deadlift, Conventional, 5 x 3 @ RPE 7-8.5
- Low Volume: 4 x 3
Lower Body Push Assistance, 3 x 6 @ RPE 6.5-8
Lower Body Pull Supplemental, 3 x 8 @ RPE 6.5-8
Lower Body Pull Isolation, 3 x 15 @ RPE 8-9.5
- High Volume only
Session 4 - Upper Body Pull
Barbell Rows, 4 x 6 @ RPE 7.5-9
Barbell Row Drop Set: 8RM, 8RM - 25%, 8RM - 50% for AMRAPs
- For High AND Medium Volume
Pull-ups, 3 x AMRAP
Speed Bench Press, 4 x 3 @ RPE 6-7.5
- High Volume: 6 x 3
Upper Body Pull Supplemental, 3 x 15 @ RPE 8-9.5
Upper Body Pull Isolation, 3 x 15 @ RPE 8-9.5
- High Volume only

Figure A-25: Block 4 Shorthand

Block 5:

Block 5
Session 1 - Squat Assessment
Back Squats, 5 x 3
- Work up to RPE 9, then back off to RPE 8
Lower Body Push Supplimental, 3 x 10 @ RPE 6.5-8
Session 2 - Bench Press Assessment
Bench Press, 5 x 3
- Work up to RPE 9, then back off to RPE 8
Upper Body Push Supplemental, 3 x 10 @ RPE 6.5-8
Standing Overhead Press, 3 x 5
- Work up to RPE 9, then back off to RPE 8
Session 3 - Deadlift Assessment
Deadlift, Conventional, 5 x 3
- Work up to RPE 8, then back off to RPE 7
Lower Body Pull Supplemental, 3 x 10 @ RPE 6.5-8
Session 4 - Accessory Assessments
Barbell Rows, 5 x 5
- Work up to RPE 8.5, then back off to RPE 7
Pull-ups, 3 x AMRAP
Upper Body Pull Supplemental, 3 x 10@ RPE 8-9.5

Figure A-26: Block 5 Shorthand

The information contained in this appendix is intended to walk you through the structure of the System. The next appendix, Appendix B, describes the template you use to plan and document your training.

Resources:

You can find an electronic copy of this program structure at: https://bruteforcestrength.com/bfs-IC/bfbss-tools/

If prompted, use username *bfbss-user* and password *bfbss-axx34s* to access this program.

Appendix B

TRAINING LOG TEMPLATES

There are two sets of templates discussed in this appendix. The first set of templates are the block templates and I'll describe each of the fields in them. The second is the training log master, where you will keep a master log of all your historical training records.

Block Templates
You can find the Microsoft Excel templates described in this appendix at the resources link at the end of this appendix.

As shown in figures B-1 and B-2 below, for each training block the templates are prepopulated with the details of the program as discussed in Appendix A. To make the most out of this template, make a copy of the template for each week's training in advance and enter specific training details (planned weight and supplemental lifts for example) for each session. Uploading the template to Google Sheets is an easy way to log your training as you lift.

Lift	Set	Planned Weight	Actual Weight	Min RPE	Max RPE	Target Reps
Back Squat	1	<RPE 8 or 85% of 1RM>		7.5	9	3
Back Squat	2	<Increase 5%>		7.5	9	3
Back Squat	3	<Increase 5% unless last set was RPE 9, then drop to RPE8>		7.5	9	3
Back Squat	4	<Increase 5% unless last set was RPE 9, then drop to RPE8>		7.5	9	3
Back Squat	5	<Increase 5% unless last set was RPE 9, then drop to RPE8>		7.5	9	3
<Pick a lower body push supplemental>	1	<Adjust to stay beetween RPE 6.5 and 8>		6.5	8	10
<Pick a lower body push supplemental>	2	<Adjust to stay beetween RPE 6.5 and 8>		6.5	8	10
<Pick a lower body push supplemental>	3	<Adjust to stay beetween RPE 6.5 and 8>		6.5	8	10
Bench Press	1	<RPE8 or 85% of 1RM>		7.5	9	3
Bench Press	2	<Increase 5%>		7.5	9	3
Bench Press	3	<Increase 5% unless last set was RPE 9, then drop to RPE8>		7.5	9	3
Bench Press	4	<Increase 5% unless last set was RPE 9, then drop to RPE8>		7.5	9	3
Bench Press	5	<Increase 5% unless last set was RPE 9, then drop to RPE8>		7.5	9	3
<Pick an upper body push supplemental>	1	<Adjust to stay between RPE 6.5 and 8>		6.5	8	10

Figure B-1: Training Block Template (left-hand columns)

Actual Reps	Actual Difficulty (RPE)	Week	Block	Training Session	Date	Training Cycle Name	Comments	Video Link
		1	Block 1 - Assessment	Session 1 - Squat Assessment		<Optional>		
		1	Block 1 - Assessment	Session 1 - Squat Assessment		<Optional>		
		1	Block 1 - Assessment	Session 1 - Squat Assessment		<Optional>		
		1	Block 1 - Assessment	Session 1 - Squat Assessment		<Optional>		
		1	Block 1 - Assessment	Session 1 - Squat Assessment		<Optional>		
		1	Block 1 - Assessment	Session 1 - Squat Assessment		<Optional>		
		1	Block 1 - Assessment	Session 1 - Squat Assessment		<Optional>		
		1	Block 1 - Assessment	Session 2 - Bench Press Assessment		<Optional>		
		1	Block 1 - Assessment	Session 2 - Bench Press Assessment		<Optional>		
		1	Block 1 - Assessment	Session 2 - Bench Press Assessment		<Optional>		
		1	Block 1 - Assessment	Session 2 - Bench Press Assessment		<Optional>		
		1	Block 1 - Assessment	Session 2 - Bench Press Assessment		<Optional>		

Figure B-2: Training Block Template (right-hand columns)

Template details:

Lift: Name the specific lift here. Lifts that are specified by the program are already entered. Choose your accessory lifts, when not specified, and enter them before heading off to the gym.

Pre-lifting mobility work and warm-up sets are not specified in the template. You may add rows and enter them if you wish.

Set #: Self-explanatory, the set number for each lift is listed.

Planned Weight: The template describes how to determine what the planned weight should be. It is good practice to populate the exact weights before hitting the gym. This allows you to calculate the planned weight and reference your master training log in advance.

Once you calculate what your planned weight should be, reference your master training log for the recent history of that lift and adjust if necessary. For example, if the program's calculations say you should be benching 315lbs, but last week you benched 225lbs at an RPE 9, an adjustment is obviously needed.

Actual Weight: Fill in the actual weight you use for each set. I find it is most effective to fill this in right after you do your set while you're resting. Filling in your results later is not only time consuming and tedious, it can be difficult to remember the specifics.

Minimum RPE: This is the lower limit of the target RPE range for the set.

Maximum RPE: This is the upper limit of the target RPE range for the set.

Target Reps: This is the target reps to complete for the set.

Actual Reps: Fill in the actual number of reps you complete for each set.

Note: I like to note if I needed spotter assistance for any reps. For example, I'll enter 3+2 if I completed three reps without help, and an additional two reps with spotter assistance. In this case the RPE will be ten because I obviously hit failure and it is likely that I need to reduce the weight for the next set.

Actual Difficulty (RPE): Enter the actual difficulty rating for the set in RPEs. If you're not familiar with how to determine RPEs, refer to Appendix E.

After you enter the set's RPE you can determine, based on the minimum and maximum planned RPEs for the set, if you should adjust the weight up or down for your next set.

Week: Update this field to identify which training week of the block (specified in the next column) you are in. When you progress to the next training block, revert back to week 1.

Note: If you are tracking your training in an overall training cycle (per the field below), you may want to use the week number based on that training cycle, versus by individual block.

Block: This field specifies which training block (1-5) you are in.

Training Session: The training session specifies which session in the training week you are completing.

Date: Enter the training date. This is important to track progress and for historical tracking.

Training Cycle Name: This is an optional field, but it is very useful if you continue using your master training log long term after you complete your first training cycle with the System. It is good to develop your own naming convention. I like to use something like <year> - <training cycle number> - <purpose>. Let's say this is your very first training cycle. The name may be '2020 – 01 – Strength Development'.

Starting with the year and an incremental number helps with sorting in your master log. If you use months in the name, I recommend using the month number for this purpose (example use 01 – January, or just 01).

Comments: Keeping robust comments helps explain things that happen during your session. For example, you are benching and didn't complete all your reps, but decide not to go down in weight because you didn't have a hand off. On your next set you get a hand off and complete all your reps successfully with an RPE of 9. Detailed comments are a great help as you plan future training sessions.

Video Link: If you capture video of your training, it is a great record of your progress. An easy way to maintain this history is to upload your videos to YouTube and record the link in your training log.

After you complete each week's training, copy the results into your training log master, as discussed below.

Training Log Master

All the effort you put in above is for naught if you don't maintain a permanent training history. I've found that it is easier to manage logging your training if your active log only contains the current week's programming. If you log your training directly into your master log, you'll quickly find yourself scrolling endlessly to get to your current training session and set.

The format of the training log master is the same as the training block templates described above. Best practice to plan and log your training is to:

- Make a copy of the training block template for the week's training.
- Customize the log for the current session. Enter the accessory lifts, copying them from the previous week if you're continuing a block. Determine the planned weights and enter them into the log. Review these targets against your actual weight from the previous week for a sanity check.
- Update any other general sections of the training log, such as the week number.
- Log your actual lifts (weight, reps, RPEs) during training.
- At the end of the week, copy all the rows from your active training log to the end of your master training log.
- Create a new active log for the following week's training.

Every effective coach will preach the importance of logging your training. The greatest strength of using this system is the ease at which you can search data. Instead of pouring through pages in your booklet to see what you benched last week, you can easily filter for a training session and/or a specific lift.

How effectively you log your training will have a direct impact on how effectively you can plan future training sessions!

Resources:

You can find an electronic copy of these templates at: https://bruteforce-strength.com/bfs-IC/bfbss-tools/

If prompted, use username *bfbss-user* and password *bfbss-axx34s* to access this program.

Appendix C

LIFT CATALOG AND SELECTING LIFTS

Appendix C: Lift Catalog and Selecting Lifts

On the resources site for the System (see the end of this appendix) I have included a catalog of the lifts I use in my programming. This list, of course, is not comprehensive. I am a fan of simplicity and the catalog shows it. You won't find one legged squats while standing on a bosu ball and balancing a 30lb dumbbell from each fingertip. You will find the basic lifts you need to get strong.

Sample excerpt from the Lift Catalog

Lift	Lift Category
Back Squat, Banded	Lower Body Push, Assistance
Back Squat, Box Squats	Lower Body Push, Assistance
Back Squat, Chains	Lower Body Push, Assistance
Back Squat, High Bar	Lower Body Push, Assistance
Back Squat, Low Bar	Lower Body Push, Primary
Back Squat, Pause	Lower Body Push, Assistance
Back Squat, Pin Squats	Lower Body Push, Assistance
Back Squat, SSB	Lower Body Push, Assistance
Barbell Rows	Upper Body Pull, Primary
Barbell Rows, Drop Set	Upper Body Pull, Supplemental
Belt Squats	Lower Body Push, Supplemental
Bench Press	Upper Body Push, Primary
Bench Press, Board Presses	Upper Body Push, Assistance
Bench Press, Chains	Upper Body Push, Assistance
Bench Press, Close Grip	Upper Body Push, Assistance
Bench Press, Dead Press	Upper Body Push, Assistance
Bench Press, Decline	Upper Body Push, Assistance
Bench Press, Double Pause	Upper Body Push, Assistance
Bench Press, Four Count	Upper Body Push, Assistance
Bench Press, Larson Press	Upper Body Push, Assistance
Bench Press, Lockouts	Upper Body Push, Assistance
Bench Press, Speed	Upper Body Push, Assistance
Bench Press, Wide Grip	Upper Body Push, Assistance
Bicep Curls	Upper Body Pull, Isolation
Box Jumps	Lower Body Push, GPP
Bulgarian Split Squats	Lower Body Push, Supplemental
Cable Rows	Upper Body Pull, Supplemental
Deadlift, Conventional	Lower Body Pull, Primary
Deadlift, Sumo	Lower Body Pull, Primary
Deadlifts, Block Pulls	Lower Body Pull, Assistance
Deadlifts, Deficit	Lower Body Pull, Assistance
Deadlifts, Pause	Lower Body Pull, Assistance
Deadlifts, Rack Pulls	Lower Body Pull, Assistance
Deadlifts, Romanian	Lower Body Pull, Supplemental
Deadlifts, Stiff-Leg	Lower Body Pull, Supplemental
Dips	Upper Body Push, Supplemental
Dumbbell Press	Upper Body Push, Supplemental
Dumbbell Press, Incline	Upper Body Push, Supplemental
Dumbbell Rows	Upper Body Pull, Assistance
Dumbbell Rows, Unsupported	Upper Body Pull, Assistance
Floor Press	Upper Body Push, Assistance
Front Squats	Lower Body Push, Supplemental
Glute-Ham Raise	Lower Body Pull, Supplemental
Goblet Squats	Lower Body Push, Supplemental
Good Mornings	Lower Body Pull, Supplemental
Good Mornings, Dead Stop	Lower Body Pull, Supplemental
Hack Squat	Lower Body Pull, Supplemental
Hip Thrusters, Barbell	Lower Body Pull, Supplemental
Incline Press	Upper Body Push, Assistance
Kettlebell Swings	Lower Body Pull, Isolation
Leg Press	Lower Body Push, Supplemental
Lunge	Lower Body Push, Supplemental
Pull-Throughs, Cable	Lower Body Pull, Isolation

Figure C-1: Lift Catalog Sample

Your primary lifts and key accessories are pre-programmed in the System. These lifts should be used as programmed unless there is a significant reason to make a substitution (for example if you have exceptionally poor shoulder mobility and need to substitute the straight bar with a safety squat bar or cambered bar for squats).

There is, however, flexibility in the selection of accessory lifts for two reasons.

- Flexibility enables you to select accessory lifts that address specific weaknesses or technical issues that you need to address.
- Changing accessory lifts from block to block stimulates additional body adaptations.

The lifts in the catalog are categorized by the muscular systems engaged and the type of lift.

Muscular System Categories: As with your training sessions, the lifts have four main categories.

- Lower Body Push – These lifts support the squat and are primarily concerned with quad strength.
- Upper Body Push – These lifts support the bench press and are primarily concerned with the pecs, anterior delts, and triceps.
- Lower Body Pull – These lifts support the deadlift, and are primarily concerned with the posterior chain, including the glutes, hamstrings, and lower back.
- Upper Body Pull – These lifts support the upper back. They are concerned with horizontal rowing and vertical pulling lifts.

Type of lift:

- Primary: This is the main movement for a lifting pattern: squat, bench press, deadlift, and overhead press. For your upper back it is the key rowing movement, barbell rows, or pulling movement, pull-ups.

  Some lifts, such as deadlifts, have more than one variation that is considered primary. For your training, the primary variation is the one you are most adept at.

- Assistance: An assistance lift uses a lifting pattern and energy system quite like the primary lift. Some examples include:

Back Squat: Pause squat, box squat, safety squat bar squat

Bench Press: Close grip bench press, wide grip bench press, Larson press

Deadlift: Snatch grip deadlift, rack pulls, block pulls, deficit deadlifts

Assistance lifts are used to emphasize a certain part of the primary lift's range of motion or to address an aspect of the primary lift's technique. They should be programmed to address weaknesses in your primary lift.

There may be times you program assistance lifts in place of primary lifts to develop your weak areas. For the purpose of this program however, you should stick with the primary as programmed.
- Supplemental: Supplemental lifts target the same muscle groups but are non-specific to the primary lift's lifting pattern and energy systems. For example, glute-ham raises strengthen the hamstrings, but the movement pattern is completely different than the deadlift. These lifts should be programmed to target weakness in your primary lift.
- Isolation: Isolation lifts are relatively low impact, single joint exercises that address a specific muscle group. Some examples include bicep curls, triceps extensions, leg extensions, and leg curls.

Resources:

You can find an electronic copy of the full lift catalog at: https://bruteforce-strength.com/bfs-IC/bfbss-tools/

If prompted, use username *bfbss-user* and password *bfbss-axx34s* to access this program.

Appendix D

ADDRESSING WEAKNESSES

This program places a great deal of emphasis on addressing your weaknesses. I created this appendix to discuss techniques and accessories that can strengthen your weak points.

Addressing Squat Weaknesses and Issues

Issue	Technique	Accessory Training	Comments
Soft rebound Soft and slow changing direction as you switch from eccentric to concentric	Attack the squat: Maintain consistent speed during descent and hit the hole with proper tempo to maximize the stretch reflex. Stay tight: Increase full body tightness and bracing, and focus on this strongly, especially at the bottom of the squat. Knee Tracking: Make sure knees track in direction of toes and hips and knees don't shift forward at the bottom.	Assistance Lifts: Speed Squats, Pause Squats, Box Squats, Parallel Pin Squats Accommodated resistance: Band Squats, Chain Squats Supplemental Lifts: Heavy Leg Press, Hack Squat to build quad strength Heavy Hip thrusters to build glute strength	Practice lifting with more confidence and explosiveness. Squat with a good speed to the bottom and push back up with as much explosiveness as possible.
Weakness at 'sticking point'	Develop an explosive rebound off the bottom of the squat to create momentum and concentrate on accelerating with all of your strength throughout the lift - keep the bar centered over your feet as you drive up out of the hole, don't let the bar shift forward. Practice bracing hard and build core strength. Don't exhale too early at the bottom of the lift, don't exhale suddenly during the lift. Slowly start snaking the air out through your teeth once you have upward momentum.	Assistance Lifts: Heavy accommodated resistance: Band Squats, Chain Squats. Accommodated resistance lifts are the best way to build strength at the sticking point. They also help train to drive upwards explosively from the bottom. Box Squats, Pause Squats, Parallel Pin Squats Explosive training: Speed Squats, Speed Deadlifts, Box Jumps, Power Cleans.	Because of mechanical leverages, the squat is naturally at its weakest just above the parallel position. At the bottom of the squat you have the aid of the stretch reflex to drive up out of the hole. As you ascend above parallel your mechanical leverages improve making the squat easier. Train to build momentum to carry you through that point and improve your ability to grind to overcome that sticking point.

Issue	Technique	Accessory Training	Comments
Issues hitting depth	Test hip mobility: Verify that you can squat through the full range of motion with proper squat technique/lifting pattern. Because individual's hip structures are different, play with your squat stance to find the stance that allows you the best hip mobility. Add hip mobility movements to your warmups. Test ankle mobility: Verify that your ankle mobility allows your knees to track properly through the full range of motion. Adjust your squat stance: Generally, a wider stance makes hitting depth more difficult due to hip mobility. However, if you have very long femurs compared to your torso, a narrow stance will force your hips backwards, causing a torso lean that brings the hips higher. A wider stance may help with depth if you have long femurs. Address torso lean: Leaning excessively brings your hips higher making depth more difficult. Keep the bar centered over your feet, don't let it drift forward. Adjust your stance to account for your femur length. If you have a proportionally short torso, consider moving the bar higher on your back. Open your hips: Turn your toes outward and spread the floor as you start your descent. Opening your hips lets them drop below parallel without pushing them backwards and leaning.	Activation and Mobilization: As you warm up, focus on movements that activate your gluteus medius/hip abductors and improve hip mobility. Banded Side Walks, Clam Shells, Banded Pause Squats (resistance bands around the knees). Assistance Lifts: Box Squats, Below Parallel Pin Squats can help you get comfortable squatting to depth and finding the proper depth. Heavy (overloaded weight/above 1RM) High Box Squats and High Pin Squats can build confidence squatting heavy weights. Supplemental Lifts: Abductor training helps build strength in the gluteus medius which helps you open your hips with heavy loads. Banded side walks, Sumo Stance Glute Bridges, Sumo Stance Hip Thrusters, Abductor Machine (low weight, high rep).	Work on building consistency with your depth, try to hit the same depth every rep and every set (not too high nor too low), regardless if it's a light warmup set or a new 1RM. Some say it takes 10,000 reps to build a pattern. Address any functional issues you have hitting depth first and find the right squat pattern for your body mechanics (foot and bar placement). Build confidence squatting all your reps to proper depth - if you can't hit depth with a heavier weight, don't put it on the bar.
Knees cave inward (knee valgus) during ascent	Test ankle mobility: Check your ankle mobility without load to verify you can squat through the full range of motion with the proper lift pattern and mechanics. If not, work on ankle mobility. Spread the Floor: As you set up and begin each rep push out against the outer edges of your shoes to engage your hip abductors and push out hard as you rebound; you should feel tightness from the outsides of your hips all the way down your legs. Adjust your stance: A wide stance increases the tendency for the knees to collapse; bring your feet in or use the 'finding your optimal stance' below. Turn your toes outward: The degree to which you turn your toes out is somewhat dependent upon your body mechanics, start with between 30-45 degrees and adjust from there. Check hip alignment: If knees come in unevenly, consider checking for structural alignment (chiropractor).	Activation and Mobilization: As you warm up, focus on movements that activate your glutes. Banded Side Walks, Clam Shells, Banded Pause Squats (resistance bands around the knees). Supplemental Lifts: Abductor training helps build strength in the gluteus medius and helps you maintain proper knee tracking during the squat. Sumo Stance Glute Bridges, Sumo Stance Hip Thrusters, Abductor Machine (low weight, high rep) Single leg training to build stabilizer strength. Lunges, Bulgarian Split Squats, Single Leg Glute Bridges If you have an issue with ankle pronation, calf training may help. Standing, slow count calf raises	Typically knee valgus, knees caving in during the ascent, is a result of your adductor strength being stronger than your abductor strength. An effective way to address this is through high volume, low intensity abductor training.

Issue	Technique	Accessory Training	Comments
Knee Valgus: Knees cave inward during descent	Adjust your stance: a wide stance increases the tendency for the knees to collapse. Bring your feet in or use the 'finding your optimal stance' below. Turn your toes outward: The degree to which you turn your toes out is somewhat dependent upon your body mechanics, start with between 30-45 degrees and adjust from there. Spread the Floor: As you set up and begin each rep push out against the outer edges of your shoes to engage your hip abductors; push out hard as you rebound. You should feel tightness from the outsides of your hips all the way down your legs. Test hip mobility: Verify that you can squat through the full range of motion with proper squat technique/lifting pattern. Because individual hip structures are different, play with your squat stance to find the stance that allows you the best hip mobility. Add hip mobility movements to your warmups. Test ankle mobility: Verify that your ankle mobility allows your knees to track properly through the full range of motion. Check hip alignment: If knees come in unevenly, consider checking your alignment (chiropractor)	Activation and Mobilization: As you warm up, focus on movements that activate your gluteus medius and improve hip mobility. Banded Side Walks, Clam Shells, Banded Pause Squats (resistance bands around the knees). Supplemental Lifts: Abductor training helps build strength in the gluteus medius which helps you maintain proper knee tracking during the squat. Sumo Stance Glute Bridges, Sumo Stance Hip Thrusters, Abductor Machine (low weight, high rep) Single leg training to build stabilizer strength. Lunges, Bulgarian Split Squats, Single Leg Glute Bridges If you have an issue with ankle pronation work on the calves. Standing, slow count calf raises	Knee valgus during the descent is often an indication that the lifter is not getting the hips to open up.
Excessive forward lean during descent	Open your hips Spread the Floor: As you set up and begin each rep, push out against the outer edges of your shoes to engage your hip abductors; push out hard as you rebound. You should feel tightness from the outsides of your hips all the way down your legs. Bar Tracking: Make sure the bar tracks in a straight line directly over the center of the lifter's feet, and does not drift forward during descent. Adjust for body mechanics Long Femurs: If lifter's femurs are proportionally long, compared to their torso, try moving their stance out to shorten their effective length. Short Torso: If the lifter's torso is proportionally short, try raising the bar to a higher position on the back.	Activation and Mobilization: As you warm up, focus on movements that activate your gluteus medius and improve hip mobility. Banded Side Walks, Clam Shells, Banded Pause Squats (resistance bands around the knees) Assistance Lifts: Box Squats, Pause Squats, Low Pin Squats: Use these as tools to ingrain the lifting pattern; make sure the bar moves in a direct line over the center of the feet through the full range of motion. Supplemental Lifts: Use lifts that build core strength as well as reinforce the proper lifting pattern. Front Squats, Zercher Squats, Goblet Squats Weighted ab training Abductor training helps build strength in the gluteus medius which helps you maintain proper knee tracking during the squat. Sumo Stance Glute Bridges, Sumo Stance Hip Thrusters, Abductor Machine (low weight, high rep)	Forward lean during the descent has a couple main causes: 1) Not opening your hips keeps you from dropping into the hole, it pushes your hips back and makes it difficult to drop below parallel. Indications of this are a more sudden forward lean as the hips near parallel. 2) Proportionately shorter torso. This is demonstrated by a more even forward lean as the lifter descends, resulting in a very flat back at the bottom of the squat, leaving the hips high.

Issue	Technique	Accessory Training	Comments
Hips shift back or rise ahead of the bar	Check for knee valgus (caving in), and review fixes for that issue. Elbows: Drive elbows forward under bar as you rebound and through the full ascent. Head Position: Pack head back into the neck and push back into the bar at the beginning of the ascent. I am not a fan of looking down in the squat. The body tends to follow the head, looking down can create the tendency to lower the chest and let the hips rise as the lifter comes up out of the hole.	Assistance Lifts: Reinforce the lifting pattern. Box Squats, Pause Squats, Low Pin Squats. Use these as tools to ingrain the lifting pattern; focus heavily on maintaining the lifting pattern at the beginning of the ascent, if the hips rise early, lower the weight; work at lower weights until the lift can be done with proper pattern. Strengthen the quads and core. Front squats, high bar close stance squats Supplemental Lifts: Strengthen the quads. Leg Press, Hack Squat Abductor training, if knee valgus contributes to the hip shift, build strength in the gluteus medius which helps you maintain proper knee tracking during the squat. Banded Side Walks, Sumo Stance Glute Bridges, Sumo Stance Hip Thrusters, Abductor Machine (low weight, high rep)	Hips shifting back and up is often caused by another issue, such as knee valgus. Address that issue first. Once that has been corrected, or if it is not the cause, look for issues with the lifter's stance, quad strength and engagement and/or core strength.
Hypermobility: Squat too deep without stretch reflex	Adjust your stance: Adjusting to a wider stance can increase tension at the bottom of the squat. Stay tight: Increase full body tightness and bracing, and focus on this strongly at the bottom of the squat	Assistance Lifts: Speed/ballistic training in squat variations, focus on a very hard rebound, consistently just below parallel. Use lifts that help build consistency in hitting proper depth. Box Squats, Pin squats, Pause Squats Supplemental Lifts: Hypertrophy: High volume, moderate weight to build muscle mass and density in the glutes and hamstrings. Romanian deadlifts, good mornings, glute-ham raises, hip thrusters	Sometimes a lifter has too much mobility, and there is no natural rebound in the squat; they can squat nearly to the floor. Squatting ultra-deep has few advantages to the lifter; maximum muscle activation and weight moved occurs generally just a couple inches below parallel. Additionally, squatting ultra-deep often leads to flexion in the lower lumbar ('butt wink'), and leads to loosening up in the hole.
Finding your optimal stance	Jump straight up as high as you can. How you land is a good starting point for your stance width	Assistance Lifts: Box Squats: With the right stance and keeping the bar in a direct line over the center of the feet, when a lifter uses the box squat, the rest of the body should naturally fall into the correct lifting pattern for the squat.	

Table D-1: Addressing weaknesses in the Squat

Addressing Bench Press Weaknesses and Issues

Issue	Technique	Accessory Training	Comments
Weak Range of Motion (ROM): Off the chest	Improve full body tightness and stability: Tighten the back by squeezing the shoulder blades together and hold them throughout the lift. Create a strong leg drive by planting your feet and pushing through the balls of your feet, push your hips horizontally toward your shoulders. Bring your chest up as you push your hips. Breath and brace by taking a big breath of air before starting each rep, tightening your core, and holding air in your chest until you have upward momentum. Leg drive is crucial as the bar reaches your chest and you start the press; don't allow your chest to soften or sink as the bar descends. Press Explosively: Regardless if the lift is 50% of your 1RM, or 105% always press every rep, even your warmups, with 110% of your power. Load the spring: Think of the bar's descent as 'loading the spring', stretching your pecs across your ribcage and stretching your triceps. Keep your back and biceps tight for stability. Bring the bar to the chest with a quick but controlled tempo and a light touch on the chest, then let that spring fire. Drive the bar upward with every muscle fiber in your body (maintain control, don't bounce the bar off your chest, keep your butt on the bench). Consistency: Touch the chest lightly and consistently in the same place every single rep.	Assistance Lifts: Lifts that emphasize the lower portion of the ROM: Spotto Press T-Shirt Press Double Pause Press 4-Count Press Lifts that increase speed and explosiveness: Speed Bench Press Accommodated Resistance (Bands and Chains) Pec-dominant lifts Wide Grip Bench Press Supplemental Lifts: Focus on lifts that emphasize the pecs and anterior delts Dumbbell Press Incline Dumbbell Press Overhead Press Strengthen your back; your back is a crucial stabilizer, it plays a huge role in helping you drive a heavy bar off your chest explosively; to help with the bench, train your back in the same plane as you press in (horizontal). Barbell Rows (heavy) Dumbbell Rows (heavy) Cable Rows (high volume) Chest Supported Rows	For raw lifters, the portion of the lift driving the bar off the chest is often a weak point. Correcting technique to get full body tightness is the number one fix for newer lifters. Strengthening the entire upper body, chest, back and shoulders, is also important, as is developing explosive speed in the lift.
Weak Range of Motion (ROM): Mid-point/upper arm parallel with the floor	Create momentum off the chest to carry through the sticking point: Work on creating an explosive drive off the chest, as noted above, to create momentum. Regardless how light the weight is, always practice accelerating the bar all the way through lockout. Never let off the acceleration because the weight is easy, or you know you've gotten it. Press the bar with 100% of your strength all the way through lockout, regardless how light or heavy it is. Note: For exceptionally light warm-ups, be careful about locking out too hard, so not to hyperextend the elbows.	Assistance Lifts: Partial ROM lifts. Use lifts that start just below the sticking point. The weak point is where bar begins to slow, not necessarily where it stops. For the bench this is usually the point where power transitions from the pecs to the triceps – strengthen this point, diminishing the size of the transition point. Floor Press Board Press (1-2 board) Pin Press (mid-range) Speed Press Accommodated Resistance (Bands and Chains)	As you press, the emphasis shifts from the pecs, delts and back to the triceps to extend/lockout the elbows. There is often a weak point (the 'sticking point') where this emphasis transitions. The pecs decline in power and the triceps ramp up. Even on successful lifts you may experience slowing, or even a slight down and up of the bar at this point before the triceps take over fully.

Issue	Technique	Accessory Training	Comments
Weak Range of Motion (ROM): At lockout	Keep your shoulders locked in place on the bench: Keep squeezing your shoulder blades together tightly as you press the bar to lockout, don't soften them and let your shoulders come up off the bench. Concentrate 100% on locking your elbows, not pushing the bar. Push yourself away from the bar. Maintain proper bar path: As you drive the bar off your chest, push slightly towards your head so the bar finishes directly over your shoulders. If you allow the bar to drift toward your feet, you will be in a terribly weak position for lockout and increase the risk of dumping the bar onto your chest.	Assistance Training Strengthen the triceps and the upper portion of the ROM: Close Grip Bench Press Floor Press Accommodated Resistance (Bands and Chains) When training partial ROM at the top end, heavily overload the weight: Board Press (3-4 board) Pin Press (top end) Supplemental Training Strengthen your triceps: Dips Tricep Extensions - there are many choices, pick your favorite, rotate them regularly (high volume)	Locking out the bar is largely a function of your triceps. However, make sure you're not 'pushing the bar up', pushing your shoulders off the bench to move the bar higher. How far you press the bar is irrelevant. The lift is over when your elbows are fully extended/locked out. Think about pushing yourself away from the bar, not pushing the bar up, then concentrate all your effort on locking your elbows.
Shoulders Push Up off the Bench	Press yourself away from the bar, then focus all your energy on locking your elbows Set your shoulders on the bench, squeeze your shoulder blades together as if you're trying to hold a quarter in place between them - don't let go of that quarter during the set.	Supplemental Training: Focus on strengthening your mid back to squeeze your shoulder blades together. Back training should be high volume, with a strong squeeze of the shoulder blades at the end of every rep: Cable Rows Chest Supported Rows (there are many choices) I like using high volume back work like this after completing heavy back work (barbell or dumbbell rows) to smoke any remaining muscle fibers in the back.	Soft shoulders during the bench is a common issue. As you press the weight, your shoulders soften, pushing upward, allowing your chest to drop. This increases the lifts ROM and makes lockout less effective.
Instability/Lack of Control at the Chest	Create full body tightness Set your shoulders on the bench, squeeze your shoulder blades together as if you're trying to hold a quarter in place between them. Use strong leg drive. Once your shoulders are planted, bring your feet back towards your hips, and drive through the balls of your feet, pushing your hips towards your shoulders, bringing your chest up as you push your hips. Breath in deeply before lowering the bar, tighten your core, and brace strongly.	Supplemental Training: Strengthen your back in the same plane as you bench - horizontally. Use a mix of high volume and high weight back training to build strength and muscle mass in the upper back. Barbell Rows, Dumbbell Rows, Chest Supported Rows, Cable Rows	Instability at the chest is often an issue with creating and maintaining full body tightness, and strength of the key bench stabilizers, back and biceps.

Issue	Technique	Accessory Training	Comments
Poor Leg Drive	Once your shoulders are set, bring your feet back towards your hips to a point where they are on the edge of discomfort. Plant your feet firmly and flat on the floor. Push through the balls of the feet, driving your hips horizontally toward your shoulders. Bring your chest up as you push your hips. This results in a small arch which builds incredible stability. If you have difficulty with the 'hip push' approach, 'heel drive' is also effective. Again, set your shoulders firmly. Bring your feet back farther under your hips until you are up on your toes and you feel tension in your lower body. Drive your heels down into the floor.		No 'dancing feet' during the bench. Unless you are isolating the chest purposely (i.e. Larson Press), failing to use leg drive in your bench negates a huge opportunity for bench press gains. Leg drive engages your entire body in the lift and creates full body tightness.
Poor Bar Path	Always start your rep and lockout with the bar directly over your shoulders. This is the most stable, powerful position to support the bar. In this position your entire muscular and skeletal system supports the bar. When you unrack, bring the bar directly to this point. The strongest touch point on the chest depends on the individual. Typically, it is between the nipple line and the base of the sternum. Once you find the strongest touch point through experimentation, hit that spot consistently with every training rep, even warm-ups. Bring the bar down quickly but controlled in a straight line from lockout to this sweet spot. When you press, push the bar slightly toward your head and directly to the lockout point over your shoulders. Do not let the bar drift toward your feet as you press, that creates an incredibly weak position and increases the chance of dumping the bar onto your chest.		
Body Instability	Your body should remain immobile as you bench, from your feet to your head. Use the techniques noted above to create full body tightness: Set your shoulders on the bench, squeeze your shoulder blades together tightly. Use strong leg drive. Breath in deeply and brace, tighten your core before lowering the bar. If your body is moving, you are leaking energy that could be used to drive the bar upward.	Supplemental Training: Strengthen your back in the same plane as you bench - horizontally. Use a mix of high volume and high weight back training to build strength and muscle mass in the upper back. Barbell Rows, Dumbbell Rows, Chest Supported Rows, Cable Rows	

Issue	Technique	Accessory Training	Comments
Bouncing/Heaving the Bar	Bouncing or heaving the bar demonstrates poor bar control and results in short term gains at best. Improving your technique and maintaining positive control of the bar through the full range of motion is the path to bigger, long term gains. Bring the bar to your chest with a quick, controlled tempo and stop on the chest with a light touch, don't sink the bar into the chest. Practice consistently using the same bar path, the same tempo, and hitting the same spot on the chest with every rep. Rule of thumb: For sets of five or less reps, bring the bar to a complete stop on the chest before pressing. Above five reps use a touch-and-go tempo.	Supplemental Training: Strengthen your back in the same plane as you bench - horizontally. Use a mix of high volume and high weight back training to build strength and muscle mass in the upper back. Barbell Rows, Dumbbell Rows, Chest Supported Rows, Cable Rows	
Shoulder Health	Bring the bar lower on the chest (nipple line or lower) to keep the elbows from flaring out which increases shoulder strain. Keep the shoulders firmly planted on the bench for every rep.	Supplemental Training: Build upper back strength to maintain shoulder position during the bench. Work on shoulder mobility before warming up for the bench. Shoulder dislocates, internal/external rotations, dead hangs, myofascial release in the pecs and anterior delts. Warm up with low weight, high rep shoulder work. Face pulls, band pull-aparts, reverse flyes.	

Table D-2: Addressing weaknesses in the Bench Press

Addressing Deadlift Weaknesses and Issues

Issue	Technique	Accessory Training	Comments
Lifting Style: Assessment	Assessment: Despite the heuristics here, the best way to determine which style deadlift is best for you is to assess both styles. Work up to a 3RM alternating sumo and conventional at each weight. One style may either allow you to lift more weight, lift the same weight more powerfully, or lift the same weight with cleaner technique. That is the style you should use as your primary deadlift approach. It is not uncommon that over time the other deadlift approach becomes stronger. Don't be afraid to change deadlift styles if it is appropriate.		There are no hard and fast rules for which style deadlift suits you better, these are general guidelines that may help decide.
Lifting Style: Conventional	Conventional: Conventional deadlifts favor a strong posterior chain, particularly a strong, healthy lower back. If your lower back, glutes and hamstrings are well trained and strong, you will have a strong conventional pull. Lifters with proportionally long arms can set up higher and more upright with a conventional deadlift, long arms may favor this style of pull.		
Lifting Style: Sumo	Sumo: Whereas conventional deadlifts are about a strong back and powerful posterior chain, sumo is about getting a strong leg drive. It is important to note that sumo deadlifts are NOT a wide stance conventional lift! Because of foot placement, conventional deadlifts push your hips back to set up. This causes you to start with a relatively horizontal back angle, particularly if you have short arms, long torso, and/or long femurs. If you do not have a comparatively strong back, this will put a lot of torque on your lower back. This may cause it to flex/round. If you have a comparatively long torso, your leverages magnify the torque on the lower back, and can make it difficult to prevent lumbar spinal flexion. If you have long femurs, a conventional stance will push your hips back farther at the start, again putting more torque on the lower back. Performed properly, a sumo stance allows you to set up with your hips closer to the bar, leaving your back in a more upright position. This reduces the lateral torque on your lower back and reduces its tendency to round. This may make sumo a better choice of deadlift style if you have: proportionally long torso, long femurs, and/or short arm span; if you have lower back issues, or lack lower back strength.		

Issue	Technique	Accessory Training	Comments
Weak Range of Motion (ROM): Off the floor	Setting Up: The key to a strong pull off the floor is a good setup. A proper setup is methodical, controlled, and efficient. It creates full body tension and facilitates a strong initial leg drive, ready to explode upward with the bar. Here are my setup Do's and Don'ts. Don't - Squat to the bar and yank it with no body tightness. - Get into the setup position and hang out there overthinking the lift. - Start with the bar forward of your center of gravity. - Roll the bar back and forth, like you've seen the big guys do on IG. Do - Tighten your upper back and pull the slack out of the bar. - Breath and brace hard to tighten your lower back and core. - Pull yourself in to the bar until you feel the weight shift onto your heels. - Keep upward tension on the bar as you pull yourself to it; focus on the building tension in your quads, glutes and hamstrings, and full body tension as you set up. - Once you reach the setup position, stop then immediately explode upward. - Attack the pull, driving down through your heels with every ounce of power in your body. - Conventional: Set up with your shins 1-2" behind the bar and knees pushed slightly over the bar to engage more quads in the initial pull. - Sumo: Set up with the bar against your shins, and your shins upright, perpendicular to the floor. - Conventional: Turn your toes out slightly for more power off the floor. - Sumo: Push your knees out to start with your hips closer to the bar. - Conventional: Pull yourself in until your shoulders are over the bar. - Sumo: Pull yourself in until your shoulders are just behind the bar.	Assistance Lifts: Emphasize the lower range of motion: Deficit Deadlifts, Snatch Grip Deadlifts Particularly if you are a conventional puller, some squat assistance lifts may help the lower end of your deadlift: Front Squats, Box Squats, Pause Squats, Pin Squats Supplemental Lifts: Strong, engaged quads help with the initial leg drive off the floor: Leg Press, Hack Squat, Front Squat, Zercher Squat A strong core helps reduce spinal flexion and transfer power to the bar: Zercher Carry, Farmer's Walk, Suitcase Carry, Loaded Plank, Back Extension	Deadlifts have no eccentric component, which, as mentioned in the bench press, 'loads the spring'. This means you get no stretch reflex to aid you in the initial portion of the pull off the floor. With a deliberate setup you can create full body tension, particularly in your quads, glutes, and hamstrings, giving you more immediate power off the floor. If your body is loose, it transfers power very inefficiently from your legs to the bar. If your body is taught like a guitar string, every muscle is engaged from your ankles to your traps. There is no flexion in your torso as you start your pull. Transfer of power from your legs, through your torso to the bar is immediate.
Weak Range of Motion (ROM): Off the floor	Rest: Fatigue has a heavy impact on deadlifts, particularly in the off the floor ROM. If you are training with heavy volume and intensity and not resting/recovering, chances are your deadlift will suffer. Lower back fatigue has a significant impact on conventional deadlifts. Hip fatigue has a significant impact on sumo deadlifts. If you're struggling with your deadlifts, and particularly if you see a huge swing in capability from week to week, consider taking steps to reduce fatigue.		

Issue	Technique	Accessory Training	Comments
Weak Range of Motion (ROM): Below the knees	Perform all lifts explosively Don't jerk the bar off the floor, but set up in a deliberate, tight manner (as described above and in my deadlift technique instructions) and initiate your pull with the maximum effort regardless what the weight is. Consciously try to accelerate through the full ROM until lockout. If you've built good power off the floor, use this explosive momentum to carry through the point just below the knees. Keep the bar close Keep the bar close to your shins and over your center of gravity through the initial stage of the ROM. If you let the bar drift out in front of your center of gravity (over or in front of your toes) your hips will come up, extending your knees and you'll lose your leg drive. To prevent this, initiate an explosive pull by driving down hard through your heels.	Explosive Training: Speed Deadlifts, Box Jumps, Power Cleans, Accommodated Resistance Deadlifts with Bands, Reverse Bands and Chains Assistance Lifts: Train the point in the ROM just below where the bar slows to a stop. Pause Deadlifts, Block Pulls, Rack Pulls Supplemental Lifts: Strong, engaged quads help with the initial leg drive off the floor, which helps build momentum: Leg Press, Hack Squat, Front Squat, Zercher Squat	A common weak point in the deadlift is for the bar to slow to a near stop just below the knees. Keep in mind, the point the bar is at its slowest is not necessarily the weak point. The weak point is where the bar begins to slow, not where it fails.
Weak Range of Motion (ROM): At lockout/above the knees	Tight Upper Back: Start the pull with your shoulders tucked down into your back pockets tightly. This facilitates the end of the lockout. As you near the top, your shoulders are already set, all you must do is stand up. Pulling with your upper back loose and shoulders forward makes lockout more challenging and pulling your shoulders back to finish the lockout is much more difficult. Leg Drive: Avoid early knee lockout, as this will end your leg drive early in the lift. Do this by driving through your heels into the floor as you start the lift - DON'T rebreak your knees once the bar crosses them. Grip: Once your grip starts to go, your body stops pulling. Tips to help your grip: Select a bar that is not bent and has good knurling. Use double overhand during warm-ups to strengthen your grip. Switch to over/under as the weight gets too heavy for double overhand. Add chalk when you can't hold the bar over/under anymore. Consider hook grip for your heaviest sets.	Assistance Lifts: Overload the top end weight. Rack Pulls, Block Pulls, Banded Deadlifts, Reverse Band Deadlifts, Chain Deadlifts - Practice rack pulls and block pulls from different heights: below the knee works the spinal erectors and posterior chain very hard to initiate the movement; above the knee allows you to greatly overload the weight	Once the bar crosses the knees, lockout is all about a strong posterior chain (glutes, hamstrings, lower back) driving your hips to lockout. A strong posterior chain can help you grind the heaviest lifts to eventual lockout. Your goal should be to lock your knees and hips at the same time.

Issue	Technique	Accessory Training	Comments
Weak Range of Motion (ROM): At lockout/above the knees	Bar Path: Keep the bar directly over your center of gravity. Don't let it swing out in front of your toes, as this creates incredibly poor leverage making the lockout more difficult; it also may cause your hips to rise resulting in your knees locking early. Grind: Don't re-tuck your knees under the bar or lean back once the bar passes your knees. Keep driving through your heels and force your hips forward. Learn to grind through to lockout. Foot Position: Arguably, turning your toes straight ahead when you set up (for conventional deadlifts) can strengthen your lockout.	Supplemental Lifts: Train the posterior chain with both heavy loads and high volume. Good Mornings - trains the spinal erectors to a greater degree, and are better for lower weights and higher volumes. Stiff Leg Deadlifts and Romanian Deadlifts - are good for heavier loads and lower volume. Note: keeping the bar close to the shins/center of gravity with Good Mornings and Stiff Leg/Romanian Deadlifts emphasizes the hamstrings; allowing the bar path to move forward of the center of gravity increases the emphasis on the lower back/spinal erectors. Glute-Ham Raises - very good hamstring isolation lift. Hip Thrusters - the best glute isolation lift. Note: for sumo pullers, more emphasis on the glutes may be more effective; for conventional pullers, use more emphasis on the hamstrings. Add in some lighter posterior chain finishers.: Cable Pull-Throughs, Kettlebell Swings, Hyperextensions, Reverse Hyperextensions Grip Training: Farmer Walks, Barbell Hold for time, Dead Hang, Pinch Grip Deadlift	
Bar rolls forward or back before leaving the floor	Set up with the bar in line with your center of gravity. As the weight gets heavy, the bar will not break the floor until it is in line with your center of gravity. Conventional: 1-2" in front of the shins, knees over the bar until shins touch, shoulders over the bar. Sumo: Shins against the bar, shins perpendicular to the floor, shoulders just behind the bar. Mobility: Lack of mobility in your upper body can make it difficult to keep the bar close to the shins. This is particularly the case with the sumo deadlift and when you use over/under grip. Your underhand arm tends to push the bar away from your body. Engage your lats to pull the bar close and keep it there. Work on your upper body mobility to allow you to set up properly with the bar close. Note: This item refers to involuntary rolling as you attempt to initiate the pull, not deliberate rolling of the bar before starting the lift…which you should never do.		

Issue	Technique	Accessory Training	Comments
Hips rise before bar leaves the floor	If you set up too low, your hips will naturally rise until you are in the optimal position for power off the floor, this is not necessarily something to be concerned about. If, however, your hips rise until your knees are near full extension, you are not getting your quads engaged, and getting little leg drive off the floor. Work on setting up by pulling yourself into the bar until you feel your weight shift to your heels, then drive through the floor with your heels. Sumo: If you are a sumo deadlifter, push your knees out hard and drive your hips forward as you start the pull.	Supplemental Lifts: Strong, engaged quads help with the initial leg drive off the floor: Leg Press, Hack Squat, Front Squat, Zercher Squat	
Lumbar Flexion	Hip Position: Allowing your hips to rotate posteriorly increases flexion in the lower back (the upper part of the hips is shifted backwards). If you have this issue, and have difficulty rotating your hips forward, work on how you set up to grab the bar. Instead of simply reaching down to grab the bar, set up like you are performing a Romanian Deadlift. Push your hips backwards, arching your back as you do, and let your chest drop as your hips go back. Keep pushing back until you can reach the bar. You can recognize this issue by an outward curve in the lower back when you grab the bar, under no load before starting the lift. Core Tightness: Work on breathing and bracing to maintain a tight core throughout the lift.	Assistance Lifts: Low weight, high volume Romanian Deadlifts; practice pushing your hips back and rotating your hips forward (arch your lower back slightly) to flatten your lower back as you do them. Supplemental Lifts: Kettlebell Swings, Cable Pull Throughs - perform them with Romanian Deadlift-like technique; push your hips back as you bring your chest down. Spinal erector training. Hyperextensions, Reverse Hyperextensions Core: Add a lot of core volume, and don't neglect weighted core work as a light finisher.	Allowing your lower back to flex/round is one of the technique issues that adds risk to the deadlift and increases the chance of lower back injury.
Thoracic Flexion	Upper Back: As you set up, pull your shoulder blades downward, hard, tucking them into your back pockets. This allows you to tighten your upper back without shortening your arm span (which would increase the lift's ROM and force you to start from a lower position, making the lift more difficult). Simply squeezing your shoulder blades together to tighten your back shortens your arm span. Pulling your shoulder blades downward also has a flattening effect on your upper back. Note: There are schools of thought that teach allowing the upper back to round and let the shoulders roll forward during deadlift setup. That is beyond the scope of this document, and not what I would recommend for newer lifters.	Supplemental Lifts: Strengthen your upper back to maintain scapula stability under heavy loads: Barbell Rows, Dumbbell Rows, Chest Supported (Machine) Rows, Cable Rows, Pull-ups, Lat Pulldowns Improve your scapular stabilization. This is done with lighter weight and higher volume: Bent-over Lateral Raise, Face Pulls, Band Pull-Aparts, Scapula Push-ups, Scapula Pull-Ups, Scapula Press-Ups. Scapula stabilization can also be done by emphasizing squeezing the shoulder blades together at the end of all rowing movements.	While thoracic, upper back, flexion/rounding is not as risky as lumbar flexlon, It still impacts the effectiveness of the lift. Strengthening the upper back helps keep the shoulders in place throughout the lift, and transfers power from the legs to the bar more effectively.

Issue	Technique	Accessory Training	Comments
Hitching	Don't lean back and tuck your knees back under the bar once it crosses your knees. This is a red light in competition and does not aid the lift or strengthen the body. From the start of the pull, drive down through your heels into the floor. This will help prevent your knees from locking early and help with leg drive through to lockout. Once the bar crosses your knees, thrust your hips forward hard, stay in position and grind to lockout. Sometimes it's better to grind and fail, than to complete a lift in a manner that does not improve strength or technique.	Supplemental Lifts: Train your glutes and hamstrings to grind through to lockout. Good Mornings, Stiff Leg Deadlifts and Romanian Deadlifts, Glute-Ham Raises, Hip Thrusters Light posterior chain finishers. Cable Pull-Throughs, Kettlebell Swings, Hyperextensions, Reverse Hyperextensions	
Soft Knees at Lockout	Don't Lean Back: The deadlift is finished when you stand up erect with your hips and knees locked out. Many lifters tend to lean back at the end to finish the lift. Leaning back does nothing for the lift and leads to soft knees, which get red lights in competition. Just stand up. Accelerate: Get in the mind set of accelerating all the way to a hard lockout for every rep. Apply max effort to every lift through the full ROM until lockout	Supplemental Lifts: Train your glutes and hamstrings to finish the lift. Good Mornings, Stiff Leg Deadlifts and Romanian Deadlifts, Glute-Ham Raises, Hip Thrusters, Glute Bridges	If you are a competitor, soft knees will result in red lights. Make sure you are fully locked out at the end of all your training reps.

Table D-3: Addressing weaknesses in the Deadlift

Resources:

You can find an electronic copy of the most current weakness assessment tables at: https://bruteforcestrength.com/bfs-IC/bfbss-tools/

If prompted, use username *bfbss-user* and password *bfbss-axx34s* to access this program.

More thorough technique reviews are available in the Brute Force Strength Book of Techniques: https://bruteforcestrength.com/bfs-book-of-techniques/

Appendix E

RPE CHARTS AND INTENSITY REFERENCE

Appendix E: RPE Charts and Intensity Reference

The RPE charts and the intensity reference table in this appendix are used to autoregulate your training, plan your training intensity, and calculate your estimated 1RM (e1RM).

RPE (Rate of Perceived Exertion) Charts

As discussed in chapter 4, RPE is used to autoregulate your training. Instead of using a static weight or percentage, using RPE allows you to go harder on days you're feeling particularly powerful, and scale back on days that you're struggling. This leads to more effective training.

The strict RPE ratings (left column) are most effective when applied to sets of five or fewer reps. RPE accuracy improves as reps per set decrease. For higher volume sets and GPP activities (farmer walks, for example), the assessment is much more subjective based on how the set *feels* (right column).

RPE	Low/Moderate Rep Range	High Volume or GPP
	Sets of 5 or less reps; judging the number of reps in the tank is easy	High rep sets or GPP activities that are not rep-based (like sled pushes or farmer walks)
10	Max Effort - either you failed to get all your reps, or you could not do one more rep	Max Effort - You are at failure; muscular and/or cardiovascular exhaustion
9.5	Near Max Effort - You possibly could do 1 more rep	Near Max Effort - You are very close to failure, muscular and/or cardiovascular
9	Very Heavy Effort - You could do 1 more rep	Very Heavy Effort - You are working very hard to complete the set; uncomfortable
8.5	Heavy Effort - You possibly could do 2 more reps	Heavy Effort - You could continue, but you are working hard to complete the set
8	Working Weight - You could do 2 more reps	Working Set - You exert effort, but can complete the set without heavy fatigue
7.5	Working Weight - You possibly could do 3 more reps	Working Weight - You exert effort, but can complete the set with light fatigue
7	Light Working Weight - You could do 3 more reps	Light Working Weight - You can complete the set with relative ease
6.5	Warm-up Weight - High end of warm-ups	Warm-up Set - You can complete the set with ease
6	Light Warm-up weight - Easy warm-up; low effort, no fatigue	Light Warm-up Set - Low effort to complete the set; no fatigue
5.5	Very low effort	Very low effort
	IMPORTANT: To 'count' in the given RPE range, a lift must be completed with competent technique (at least 80% correct)	

Rules:
1. When your RPE exceeds the maximum on your first set but is doable with correct form, try to complete a second set before lowering the weight. You'll find at times it takes a set at your working weight to get your CNS and technique really dialed in.
2. If the weight is at or below the minimum RPE rating, complete at least three sets before raising the weight. Make sure you will be able to complete all your sets and reps in your latter sets as fatigue sets in.
3. If the weight is at or below the minimum RPE rating, but it will be progressing higher with each set, follow the plan, don't leapfrog planned weight increases.

4. When adjusting the weight up or down, start with a five percent change in weight.

Note: These rules apply to the primary lifts for a session; adjust as necessary for accessory work.

Table E-1: RPE Reference Tables

Always keep in mind that the RPE ratings are subjective measures. For the best results, don't over analyze your ratings. Trust your instincts. Your skill at assessing lifts' difficulty will improve with experience and as you learn your capabilities.

RPE Intensity Reference Chart

Reactive Training Systems (https://www.reactivetrainingsystems.com) has developed a generalized chart that correlates the *number of reps per set* and a *specific RPE rating* to the percentage of your current 1RM (or e1RM).

- This is a generalized chart. The intent is to hit the ballpark of your target training intensity given the number of reps per set. Because every person is different (Law of Individual Differences), your actual training intensity is often a bit above or below that specified in the chart.
- The chart's accuracy improves as the repetitions decrease or the RPE rating increases. This is because lower reps and/or higher RPEs leave less room for subjectivity.
- I've found this chart is effective for estimating the starting weight for a training session. After calculating a target weight, compare it against the previous week's results and adjust if necessary.
- The RPE intensity reference chart is intended only for use with primary lifts (squat, bench press, deadlift, overhead press).

For the System, the planned starting weight/intensity is specified for the training block. Appendix A lists the staring percentage for each block. It is also copied into the training log templates. The RPE intensity reference chart will be used, however, to calculate your e1RMs for each training session. Appendix F describes how to use this chart and calculate your e1RM.

		Reps											
		1	**2**	**3**	**4**	**5**	**6**	**7**	**8**	**9**	**10**	**11**	**12**
RPE	**10**	100%	95.50%	92.20%	89.20%	86.30%	83.70%	81.10%	78.60%	76.20%	73.90%	70.70%	68%
	9.5	97.8	93.9	90.70%	87.80%	85.00%	82.40%	79.90%	77.40%	75.10%	72.30%	69.40%	66.70%
	9	95.50%	92.20%	89.20%	86.30%	83.70%	81.10%	78.60%	76.20%	73.90%	70.70%	68.00%	65.30%
	8.5	93.90%	90.70%	87.80%	85.00%	82.40%	79.90%	77.40%	75.10%	72.30%	69.40%	66.70%	64.00%
	8	92.20%	89.20%	86.30%	83.70%	81.10%	78.60%	76.20%	73.90%	70.70%	68.00%	65.30%	62.60%
	7.5	90.70%	87.80%	85.00%	82.40%	79.90%	77.40%	75.10%	72.30%	69.40%	66.70%	64.00%	61.30%
	7	89.20%	86.30%	83.70%	81.10%	78.60%	76.20%	73.90%	70.70%	68.00%	65.30%	62.60%	59.90%
	6.5	87.80%	85.00%	82.40%	79.90%	77.40%	75.10%	72.30%	69.40%	66.70%	64.00%	61.30%	58.60%

Source: *Chart adopted from Reactive Training Systems, RTS, https://www.reactivetrainingsystems.com*

Figure E-1: RPE Intensity Reference

Training Weight Percentages

As mentioned, for this system you will use the training percentage listed in Appendix A for your training sessions. Since this program is for newer lifters, I have adjusted the percentages slightly from this chart. For example, for Block 1, Session 2 Bench Press, the weight for your first set will be 75% of your current e1RM. If, however, you were using this RPE Intensity Reference to determine the weight for set 1 you would use:

- Five Reps
- RPE (minimum) 7
- 78.6% of your e1RM – which is the intersection of five reps and 7 RPE

For subsequent sets you will adjust the training weight to stay above the minimum RPE rating for the set (7), and below the maximum RPE rating for the set (8.5).

Estimated 1RM

After completing your training session, you will use this chart to calculate your weekly e1RM for the primary lifts (I suggest using e1RM only for squat, bench press, deadlift, and overhead press). Use training history and RPE guidelines for determining training weights for other lifts and accessories.

To determine your e1RM, first you must determine which set to base it on. Use your strongest working set. This is the set that:

- Uses the heaviest weight.
- Has the most reps at that weight.

- Has the lowest actual RPE rating for that weight and number of reps.

I have created a simple calculator to find your e1RM, as described in Appendix F. To calculate the e1RM you will need the weight, reps, RPE from your strongest working set. Find the reps along the top axis and the RPE rating along the left axis corresponding with your lift. The intersection of these is the intensity percentage you will use. To calculate your e1RM based on that set, you can use the calculator discussed in Appendix F, or use the formula: Weight / Intensity Percentage.

For example:
- Your top set was 100kg x 3 reps at RPE 8
- The relative intensity of this set is 3 reps at RPE 8, 86.3%
- Your e1RM is 100kg / .863 = 115.9kg

Remember that these calculations are generalized, and there will be some margin of error. However, given the formula considers not just the weight and reps, but also the RPE of the set, the accuracy will be a better representation of your current capability than the simple online 1RM calculators.

Resources:
You can find an electronic copy of the most current RPE charts and intensity reference table at: https://bruteforcestrength.com/bfs-IC/bfbss-tools/
   If prompted, use username *bfbss-user* and password *bfbss-axx34s* to access this program.

References:
The RPE Reference Table and RPE Intensity Reference chart are adopted from Reactive Training Systems at: https://reactivetrainingsystems.com

Appendix F

ESTIMATED 1RM (e1RM) AND PLANNED WEIGHT CALCULATOR

To help you plan and track your training, the System includes a calculator to help find your e1RM and planned weights. You can download the calculators from the link in the resources section below. This appendix describes how to use them.

e1RM Calculator

	Weight Lifted	Reps	RPE	RPE Intensity %	E1RM	Comments
						Estimated 1RM (E1RM)
==>						1. Determine your strongest lift for the session. It is the set with the highest weight, most reps at that weight, and lowest RPE rating. 2. Enter the weight, reps, and RPE rating for that set into the chart. 3. Find the % for that rep and RPE rating on the RPE Intensity Reference chart and enter it. 4. Your E1RM for that lift will be calculated.
					0	
Example	100	4	9.5	87.80%	113.8952	
					Weight / %	

Figure F-1: e1RM Calculator

To find your current e1RM, the you must first determine your 'strongest' set. I've created rules to determine which working set to use:

- Select set with the highest weight.
- At that weight, pick the set with the most reps.
- At that weight and reps, pick the set with the lowest RPE.

Note that your first set is not always your strongest set.

To calculate your e1RM:

- Enter the weight, reps and RPE rating into the e1RM calculator. The Reps and RPE are for record keeping – they are not used in the calculation.
- Using the Reps and the RPE rating you've entered, look up the RPE Intensity % from the RPE Intensity Reference chart in appendix E.
- Once you enter the percentage from the reference chart, it will calculate your e1RM.

This is an estimate based on a generalized chart. Everyone has individual differences which will affect its relative accuracy. Accuracy is also affected by the number of repetitions and RPE rating of your set. Lower rep sets and higher RPE ratings usually lead to a more accurate estimate.

You will use your e1RM to plan future training. It is important to track it so you can refer to it for planning, and to track your progress. Once you've calculated your e1RM, record it into your metrics log. The metrics log is described in Appendix I.

Planned Weight Calculation						
	Min RPE	Target Reps	RPE Intensity %	E1RM	Planned Weight	Comments
==>						1. Enter the target reps and minimum RPE for the set 2. Enter the % for that Rep/RPE combo from the RPE Intensity Reference 3. Enter your current E1RM for the lift 4. Your planned starting weight will be calculated.
					0	
Example	7	5	78.6%	125.0	98.25	
					Weight x %	

Figure F-2: Planned Weight Calculator

The planned weight calculator is in the same worksheet. You use it much the same way you used the e1RM calculator. The formula, however multiplies the RPE Intensity Percentage by your current e1RM to determine the planned working weight.

To use this calculator:

- Enter the minimum RPE for your first working set, as listed in your training program (see the note below).
- Enter the target repetitions for your first working set.
- Refer to the RPE Intensity Reference Chart in appendix E to find the RPE Intensity Percentage for that RPE and number of repetitions. Enter that percentage.
- Enter your current e1RM from your metrics log.
- Once you've entered your e1RM, it will calculate the planned weight for your first working set.

Note: For the System, your starting weight percentage is given in each of your training sessions (see appendix A). Plug the percentage from appendix A into the column for RPE Intensity Percentage.

It is always good practice to compare the planned weight with the recent results in your training log. Based on your training log (weight lifted, reps completed, RPE ratings), you may want to adjust the planned weight for the current week's training. You should target hitting the low end of the RPE range for the first set. During training you will adjust the weight as necessary to stay within the RPE ranges.

Resources:
You can find an electronic copy of these calculators at: https://bruteforce-strength.com/bfs-IC/bfbss-tools/

If prompted, use username *bfbss-user* and password *bfbss-axx34s* to access this program.

Appendix G

RPE AND INTENSITY ADJUSTMENTS

Not all lifts are the same. The RPE Intensity Reference chart in Appendix E applies most directly to the squat, the bench press, and the deadlift. When using it to plan weights for other lifts, you will need to make some adjustments. Some lifts are more difficult, and you will need to bring the intensity down. Some lifts are less difficult, and you will want to increase the intensity.

I've developed this chart to provide some general guidelines for these adjustments.

Lift/Type	Adjustment	Rationale/Comments
Squat, Safety Squat Bar (SSB)	-10%	Squatting with the SSB is more challenging than a back squat due to the leverages and mechanics involved. Keep in mind that an SSB bar typically weighs more than a standard power bar, so make sure you know your bar's weight.
Speed Sets (Squat, Bench Press, Deadlift)	-20%	For speed squats, bench press, and deadlift; speed work is meant to maintain high bar speed and explosive movements. The weight needs to be kept lighter than typical working sets. If the bar begins to slow, either reduce the reps, or reduce the weight.
Squat, Zercher	-20%	Zercher squat, like front squats, are more challenging due to the leverages and mechanics involved.
Squat, Box/Pin/Pause	-10%	Reduce the weight due to reduced assistance from the stretch reflex, due to the dead stop. As the pause increases from two to seven seconds, you may need to reduce the weight more.
Chains	+10%	Top end weight (bar weight plus total chain weight) is 10% above weight used for straight bar weight at the given lift. Chains should make up about 25% of the total top end weight.
Bench Press, Slingshot	+10%	If slingshot 1RM/e1RM is unknown, add 10% to your normal bench press weight. It is a better strategy to track the 1RM/e1RM of your slingshot assisted bench.
Squat, Wraps	+10%	If 1RM/e1RM for squats with wraps is unknown, add 10% to your normal squat weight. It is a better strategy to track the 1RM/e1RM of your wrapped squats.
Partial ROM	Use RPE	Partial ROM lifts will need to be based on the RPE of the lifts. There are too many variables for each individual to judge this. For example, a partial ROM lift that starts at the sticking point may be more difficult than a full ROM lift.
Deadlift, Deficit	-10%	Because of the lower starting point of the lift, and the lengthening of the ROM, the lift becomes more challenging. This includes Snatch Grip Deadlift, which in effect lengthens the ROM.
Bench Press, Close Grip	-10%	For most lifters, the increased length of the ROM, and the shift in emphasis to the triceps and anterior delts reduces the weight you can lift.
Bench Press, Floor Press	-10%	Because of the dead stop, and the dead stop being at the common sticking point in the bench press, floor presses can be more challenging than full ROM lifts.
Bench Press, Board Press	+5% per Board	Each board reduces the lift's ROM; since it is not a dead stop, the use of stretch reflex remains to assist the lift.
Squats, Front Squats	-25%	Front squats are more challenging than back squats, due to the difficulty supporting the bar in the front rack position, and the leverages/mechanics involved.
Stiff-Leg Deadlift (SLDL) / Romanian Deadlift (RDL)	-25%	Due to the emphasis placed on the lower back, and the reduced leg drive in the lift, SLDLs and RDLs are more challenging than normal deadlifts.
Dumbbell Press	-65%	Because of the significant decrease in stability when pressing dumbbells versus pressing a bar, dumbbell presses are more challenging than barbell presses. Total weight used is less than barbell weight (for each dumbbell; for example if the bar weight would be 100lbs, use 35lb dumbbells).
Dumbbell Press, Incline	-70%	Because emphasis shifts from your pecs to your anterior delts, incline dumbbell presses are typically more challenging than flat dumbbell presses.

Lift/Type	Adjustment	Rationale/Comments
Squats, High Bar	-10%	Depending on individual body mechanics, leverage when performing high bar squat is typically less advantageous than low bar squats. Note that if your body mechanics favor high bar, or if you are more practiced with the high bar squat, this may actually be a stronger lift.
Deadlift Rack Pulls/Block Pulls	Use RPE	Because of the nature of rack pulls, estimating an adjustment is very challenging: If starting below the knee, you can use less leg drive than from the floor, and the starting point places significant emphasis on your lower back. This may make them more challenging than full ROM deadlifts. If starting above the knee, typically you can lift a great deal more than full ROM deadlifts - these should be used for weight overload training. Note: Keep in mind that Rack Pulls/Block Pulls often start very slowly, be patient with them at the beginning - don't quit on the lift if it takes a moment to get started.
Bench Press, Pin Press	Use RPE	Because of the nature of pin presses, estimating an adjustment is very challenging: With the pins set from just above the chest to the sticking point (around mid-ROM), due to starting from a dead stop, they will be more challenging than a full bench, or board press, which gains advantage from the stretch reflex. With the pins set above the sticking point you should be able to lift a great deal more than full ROM bench presses - these should be used for weight overload training. When using Pin Presses above the sticking point for overload, I like to start with a weight based on RPE, and subsequently increasing the weight each set until I hit failure. Note: Keep in mind that presses often start very slowly, be patient with them at the beginning - don't quit on the lift if it takes a moment to get started.
RPE Planning Guidelines		Below are some guidelines I use when planning what the target RPEs should be
Strength Training	RPE 7 - 8.5	I use RPE 7 to RPE 8.5 as the training range when my goal is to build the strength foundation. My target is to start at a weight that results in an RPE 7, and progress upward in weight as sets progress, keeping the RPE at or below RPE 8.5. Keep in mind that the RPE will rise not only with the weight, but also with fatigue as you get deeper into the sets. Typical training range for strength is 3-6 reps.
Strength Training - Deadlifts	RPE 6.5 - 8	Because deadlifts create a heavy fatigue toll on every system in the body, I train it at a lower intensity than other lifts. In addition to slightly lower RPE, I often use a slightly higher rep range as well, to keep the intensity down. For example, when using singles for squats and bench press, I'll use triples for deadlifts, unless in a competition cycle. Typical training range for strength is 3-6 reps.
Power Training	RPE 7.5 - 9	I use RPE 7.5 - 9 when training for power. Again, select a starting weight for the first working set that will be at the low end of the range, and keep the weight below the top end of the range as the sets progress. Training range for power development is 1-3 reps.
Power Training - Deadlifts	RPE 7 – 8.5	As with strength training, deadlifts should be trained at a slightly lower intensity.

Lift/Type	Adjustment	Rationale/Comments
Hypertrophy Training	RPE 6.5 - 8	Start with weights at the lower end of the RPE range and keep the RPE under the top end of the range as the sets progress.
Speed Training	RPE 6 - 7	Intensity for speed training should be kept low, and focus should be on bar speed as well as the RPE range. If the bar speed or explosiveness of the lift wanes, the weight should be reduced.
Machine Training	RPE + 1	When training with machines, I typically push the intensity up in the RPE scale. For instance, if using leg press for strength, I'll increase it to RPE 8-9.5. Because of the controlled movements and their isolation effect, you can typically train at a higher intensity with machines with a lower impact on overall fatigue.
Restoration / Recovery / Ramp-up Cycles	RPE -10 to 20%	When in a restoration or recovery cycle between heavy development cycles, I bring the intensity down. Typically, I set the starting weight at the RPE appropriate for the training approach, and then reduce the weight by 10%. I use ramp-up cycles when a lifter hasn't trained for a while. Week 1 I set the starting weight based on the appropriate RPE and reduce it by 20%. Week 2 I reduce it by 10%.

Table G-1: RPE and Intensity Adjustments

As with planning your primary lifts, this chart is a guideline to help plan your starting lifts. To apply it:

- Look up the target intensity, by referring to the RPE Intensity Reference Chart in Appendix E. Multiply the percentage from the chart by your e1RM.
- Apply the adjustment from table G-1 to the planned weight. For example, for Safety Squat Bar squats, reduce the planned weight by ten percent.
- Refer to your master training log and look up what weight you have used most recently for the lift. Review the weight used, number of reps, and actual RPE resulting from that recent lift. Adjust your starting weight if necessary.
- Adjust the weight as necessary during training to remain within the RPE guidelines for your plan.

Example:

Your training plan lists Safety Squat Bar Squats, 3x5 at RPE 7-8.5. Your Squat e1RM is 500lbs.

- Look up the target intensity for the first set, using 5 reps at RPE 7 (you want to start at the low end of the RPE scale) – 78.6%.

- Multiply your e1RM by 78.6% - 393lbs.
- Since Safety Squat Bar Squats are typically tougher than Back Squats, use the adjustment from this table, -10% - 353.7lbs. If you're using lb plates, round to 355 for your set. If you're using kilo plates round to 352.7lbs/160kg.

Resources:

I maintain updates to this table as I come across new information. You can find an electronic copy of the latest table at: https://bruteforcestrength.com/bfs-IC/bfbss-tools/

If prompted, use username *bfbss-user* and password *bfbss-axx34s* to access this program.

Appendix H

ASSESSMENT LOG

As you have likely gathered through the course of this book, logging is critically important to progress. The assessment log is particularly important. It forces you to think about what your weaknesses are and how to address them. You will use this information to tailor your training. This little nuance is one of the strengths of the System.

How to use the log

Most of this System is numbers based. When you're doing your assessments, get wordy for best results. The more you write here, the better. It is a great reference as you move from block to block, and it helps keep your focus on what you need to improve.

The log is set up to measure your primary lifts as you progress through each block. Feel free to add additional lifts that you would like to assess. As you finish each block (or if something significant occurs during a block), take notes of the following information:

- e1RM: Note your final e1RM at the end of the block; this will help you measure objective progress.
- Weak ROM: What is the weakest point in your lifts? Off the chest in

the bench press? At the sticking point in the squat? Locking out the deadlift? Noting where your lift is weak helps you determine which accessory lifts will make the most impact on your lift. It may also help you identify points in your technique to focus on.

- Technique Issues: Assess each lift's technique critically. Don't be shy to have an experienced lifter observe your lifts and give you feedback. Be descriptive in your assessment. Do your knees cave in when you squat? Are you hitching your deadlifts?

- Injuries: Make note of any injuries, whether pre-existing or new. Include mobility issues. Use this information to determine if you need to adjust your program. *If you have injuries, do consult a physician to make sure you can continue lifting safely!*

	Block 1	Block 2	Block 3	Block 4	Block 5
Squats:					
E1RM					
Weak ROM					
Technique Issues					
Injuries					
Bench Press:					
E1RM					
Weak ROM					
Technique Issues					
Injuries					
Deadlift:					
E1RM					
Weak ROM					
Technique Issues					
Injuries					
Overhead Press:					
E1RM					
Weak ROM					
Technique Issues					
Injuries					

Figure H-1: Assessment Log

After completing your assessment, refer to Appendix D for assistance in addressing them.

Resources:

You can find an electronic copy of this log template at: https://bruteforce-strength.com/bfs-IC/bfbss-tools/

If prompted, use username *bfbss-user* and password *bfbss-axx34s* to access this program.

Appendix 9

METRICS LOG

Your metrics log is, in my opinion, the second most important log, following your master training log. In this log you will track your training weeks' results and capture your e1RMs. This detail will be used to plan future training. For each primary lift you will log:

- Date: Use the first day of the training week. I use Sundays for this date.
- Weight: Identify the strongest set for the lift as described in Appendix F. Enter the weight for that set.
- Reps: For the set identified enter number of reps completed.
- RPE: Enter the actual RPE rating for the identified set.
- e1RM: Using the calculator described in Appendix F, enter the e1RM for the set.

The training log has calculations to identify changes from week to week. It also calculates the total of your squat, bench press and deadlift e1RMs, and week to week changes in your total. You can use the changes in this log do determine when it is appropriate to end one block and move to the next.

- *Best e1RM Total*: As you progress, plug in your best total in this column. This helps track where you are in comparison to your strongest week.
- *Injuries*: Log any injuries or physical issues you encounter during the week (including fatigue and external factors affecting your training). This can help account for changes in your lift results.
- *Training Block*: List the name of the training block. This will help you measure your results, block to block.
- *Comments*: If there are any additional notes you feel help characterize your training week, enter them here. This can be important information when you assess your block at the end.

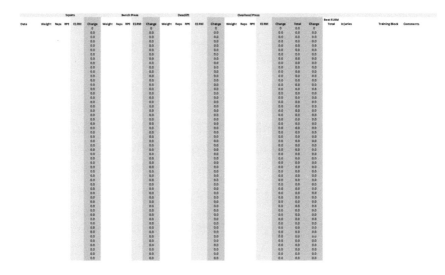

Figure I-1: Metrics Log

Resources:
You can find an electronic copy of this log template at: https://bruteforce-strength.com/bfs-IC/bfbss-tools/

If prompted, use username *bfbss-user* and password *bfbss-axx34s* to access this program.

Appendix J

LIST OF FIGURES

Chapter 2:

Appendix A:

Appendix H:
- Figure H-1: Assessment Log

Appendix I
- Figure I-1: Metrics Log

ABOUT THE AUTHOR

Ken Gack 'the Ripper' has spent over three decades under the bar, with over two of those decades on the powerlifting platform. In this time, he has competed in over 50 powerlifting competitions and has coached powerlifters and strength athletes for over a decade. He has racked up a long list of accomplishments in the sport of powerlifting.

- Former International Powerlifting Federation World Champion and has competed in the world championships ten times.
- Competed in the Arnold Sports Festival, one of the biggest sporting events in the world, three times, including one appearance in Europe.
- Six-time USA Powerlifting National Champion.
- Member of the Washington State Powerlifting Hall of Fame.
- Has held USA Powerlifting State and American records in the squat, bench press, deadlift and total.
- Has coached dozens of powerlifters in competition at the local, state, national, and world level.
- Has developed an extensive on-line library of strength training and lifting articles and materials.

Ken has established his own unique style of strength training through lifting and studying under some of the best coaches in the world, decades of personal competition experience, and planning and coaching his lifters through hundreds of thousands of sets of training. He has distilled this experience and approach into the Beginner's Strength System described in this book.

CPSIA information can be obtained
at www.ICGtesting.com
Printed in the USA
BVHW022053061220
594968BV00005B/28